STRENGTH ISN'T BORN, IT'S FORGED IN THE BROKEN.

WIN BROKEN

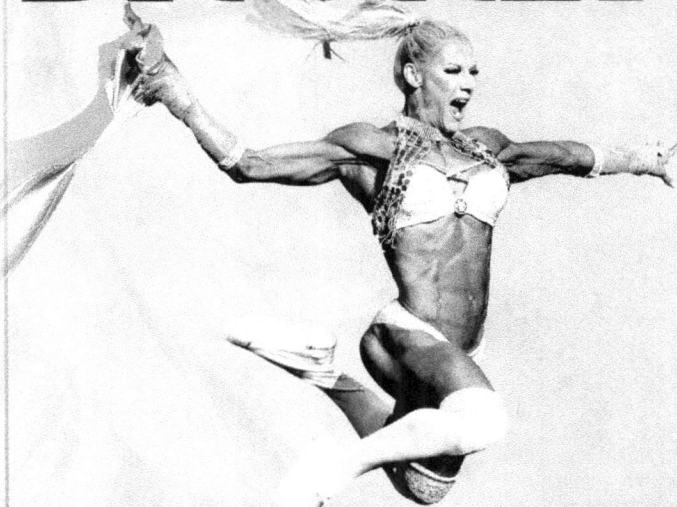

WHITNEY JONES

3X MS FITNESS OLYMPIA ~ IFBB FITNESS PRO ~ ENTREPRENEUR

EMPOWERINGLEGENDS.COM

Win Broken

Strength Isn't Born, It's Forged In The Broken

Whitney Jones

WE HELP
AUTHORS

WeHelpAuthors.com

Win Broken

Copyright © 2025 by Whitney Jones

2025 Whitney Jones ™

2025 We Help Authors ™

2025 Empowering Legends ™

ISBN#: 979-8-9904792-3-4 Paperback

ISBN#: 979-8-9904792-4-1 Hard Cover

ISBN#: 979-8-9904792-5-8 Audiobook

Printed in the United States of America

For bulk orders, please visit: **WeHelpAuthors.com/bulk**

DEDICATION

To my mom, the strongest, most determined woman I've ever known—your grit, tenacity, and endless compassion taught me that the greatest treasure in life is found in how we care for others. You left too soon, but your legacy of selflessness and love will always be my compass.

To my dad, who showed me that a rich life isn't about money but about living with joy, humor, and connection. Your dad jokes (even now, in the haze of dementia) are timeless treasures, and your infectious smile still lights up every room.

To my boys, Brody and Jake, my pride, my joy, and the reason for my six-pack abs—thanks to all the laughter you've given me over the years. Watching you grow and navigate life has been my greatest adventure. I hope our wild, crazy, love-filled journey has armed you with lessons to create your own extraordinary lives.

And to *you,* the person holding this book: buckle up—I'm about to become the best friend you never knew you needed. Let's laugh, cry, and conquer life together. With Love, Whitney

CONTENTS

How to Use This Book

Look, I get it—life is messy, time is short, and you've got about a million things competing for your attention right now. So let me tell you exactly how to get the most out of this book (because if you're going to invest your precious time with me, I want to make it count).

First of all, this isn't your typical "read it cover-to-cover" kind of book. Think of it more like having a conversation with your slightly rowdy (but wise) best friend who's been through it all and lived to tell the tales. Here's how to make it work for you:

If You're Short on Time

- Each chapter stands alone, so feel free to jump to what you need most right now

- Look for the "Your Turn" sections at the end of each chapter for quick, actionable steps

- Use the Notes pages to jot down ideas that hit home (because trust me, you'll want to remember these)

If You're Going All In

- Grab a pen—this is a workbook as much as it's a book

- Don't skip the exercises (they're not fillers, they're game-changers)

- Share your journey—use **#WinBroken** on social media to connect with others

- Keep your sense of humor handy—we're going to need it

What You'll Find Inside

- Real stories (sometimes embarrassingly real)

- Practical strategies (that actually work)

- Action steps (because reading without doing is like watching someone else eat a cookie)

- Space for reflection (because your journey matters too)

Remember: This book isn't about being perfect—it's about being perfectly okay with being imperfect. So whether you read it front to back, skip around, or just flip to whatever page the universe guides you to, you're doing it right.

Now, let's go win broken together.

—Whitney

Foreword

Dancing Through Life's Red Lights

By Dave Streen

WeHelpAuthors.com/dave

I was driving early one morning, barely awake, because I hadn't had my coffee yet. Now, I'm serious about my coffee, and the Bulletproof Coffee at Genius Network is my favorite. But I can't have coffee at home *and* again at Genius, or I'll be up all night. So, half-awake, I found myself at a stoplight, glancing around, trying to shake the sleepiness, when I saw this blonde woman in a custom purple Porsche, just dancing her heart out to the music. She was completely in her own world, and I thought, *now that's someone who really lives.*

As the light turned green, she sped off, and wouldn't you know it, we were headed to the same place. When we parked and got out around the same time, I saw it was Whitney Jones, the three-time Ms. Fitness Olympia Champ. She walked into the building just ahead of me, and even though she wasn't dancing now, she might as well have been—she had this energy that was contagious, almost like her entire life had a soundtrack she was moving to.

Inside, I got to witness something special. Picture Norm from *Cheers,* where everyone yells his name when he walks in—well, Whitney's entrance was like that, only on a whole other level. As soon as she walked in, people lit up, like they'd been waiting just for her. They didn't just call out her name; they jumped up, ran over to hug her, and brought this whole new level of energy into the room. Watching that, I realized this woman wasn't just a powerhouse on stage; she had this rare ability to elevate everyone around her at all times.

Now, you might see someone like Whitney and think she's got it all together, that life must be perfect. But here's the thing: I know people, and I know that nobody is immune to life's struggles. Everyone's got something—a challenge with health, finances, relationships, you name it. We're all a bit broken in one way or another. Whitney, though, has this incredible gift of embracing life fully, cracks and all, and still showing up as the best version of herself.

In this book, Whitney reveals the blueprint for how to keep moving forward, even when life isn't perfect, how to stay relentless, and how to find your power, no matter what you're up against. She's going to show us all how to win—even when broken.

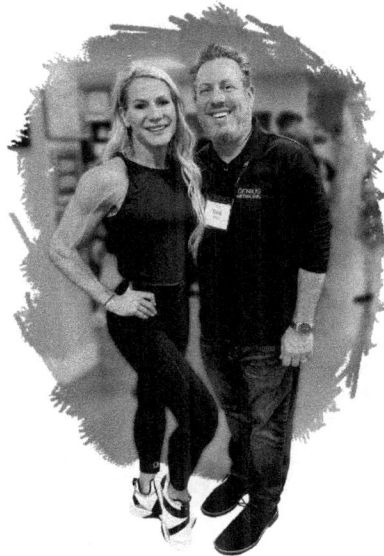

$P_{RELUDE:}$

The Whitney I Know

By Ashley Garcia
Business Partner, Partner-in-Crime, Past Client, and Friend

How do you capture the essence of someone who defies gravity with her laugh, resets broken bones like they're Lego pieces, and turns every moment—even panic-stricken ocean adventures—into a lesson in living fully? After a decade of friendship and business partnership with Whitney Jones, I can tell you it's not easy. But let me try to show you the Whitney I know, the one behind the three Olympia titles and successful businesses. The one whose real superpower isn't her physical strength, but her golden heart.

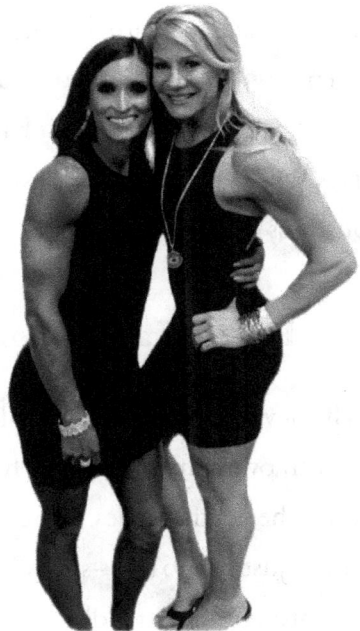

Whitney and Ashley

The Laugh That Defies Gravity

If you've ever been in the same room as Whitney, you've heard it—that infectious laugh that bounces off walls and comes with a signature lean-back motion and an involuntary slap to whoever's standing closest. It doesn't matter if you have no idea what's funny; you'll find yourself laughing too. From eight-year-old dad jokes to perfectly timed "That's what she said" moments, Whitney turns every situation into an opportunity for joy.

We've had countless nights where we should have been working but ended up literally rolling on the floor laughing instead. During our 2024 fitness challenge with 80 entrepreneurs, our Monday Zoom calls became legendary—not just for the valuable content, but for Whitney's spontaneous dance breaks and our barely contained giggles. Who else can change lives while making their best friend try not to pee their pants during a business call?

The Heart of a Champion

Whitney's strength isn't just about the weights she can lift or the injuries she can overcome. It's about how fiercely she fights for others, even while facing her own battles. When I was training for my IFBB pro card, she wasn't just my coach—she was my cornerstone. For two years, she guided me through every roadblock and challenge. When I finally won, she was the second person I hugged (after my husband), and we both cried like we'd won the lottery.

But here's what makes Whitney special: she brings that same level of investment to everyone she meets. Whether you're a client, friend, or stranger, she wants your success as much as her own. It's not strategy; it's just who she is.

The Magic of Motherhood

Want to see Whitney's real superpowers? Watch her with her boys. As a single mom, she's mastered being the taxi driver, chef, cheerleader, provider, and strength of her family—all while building an empire and collecting world titles. But what truly amazes me is how she never lets life's challenges dim their light.

This summer in Cabo, I watched Whitney—who's terrified of the ocean—climb down a boat ladder into deep water, stealing everyone's safety noodles and breathing like she needed a paper bag, all because her boys wanted to go snorkeling. What she didn't see was their eyes sparkling with pride and joy, not because she was perfect, but because she showed up, tried, and made them laugh through it all.

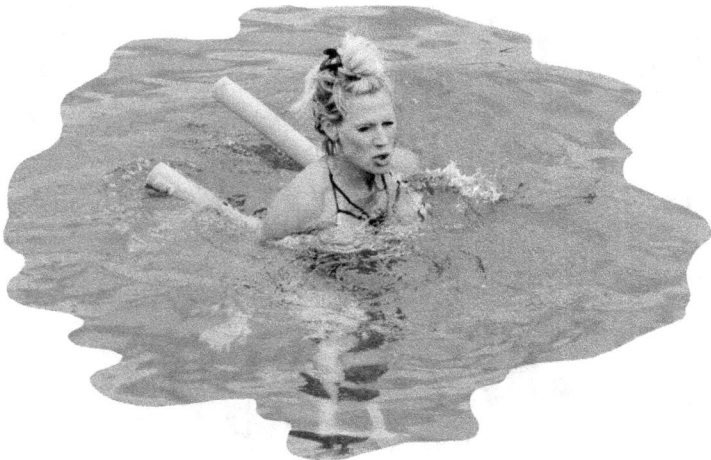

The Ultimate Winning Broken Story

Success is often measured in titles, trophies, and bank accounts. But watching Whitney navigate life—whether she's coaching clients, parenting her boys, or attempting to befriend fish in the ocean—I've learned that true success is about showing up authentically, laughing through the chaos, and lifting others while you climb.

In this book, you'll read about Whitney's incredible achievements, her comebacks from injuries, and her strategies for winning broken. But as you turn these pages, remember this: behind every triumph and face plant is a woman who leads with her heart, laughs from her soul, and proves that being perfectly imperfect is the most powerful way to live.

Whitney Jones isn't just a champion athlete or successful entrepreneur—she's a force of nature wrapped in glitter, grit, and dad jokes. And I'm proud to call her my friend.

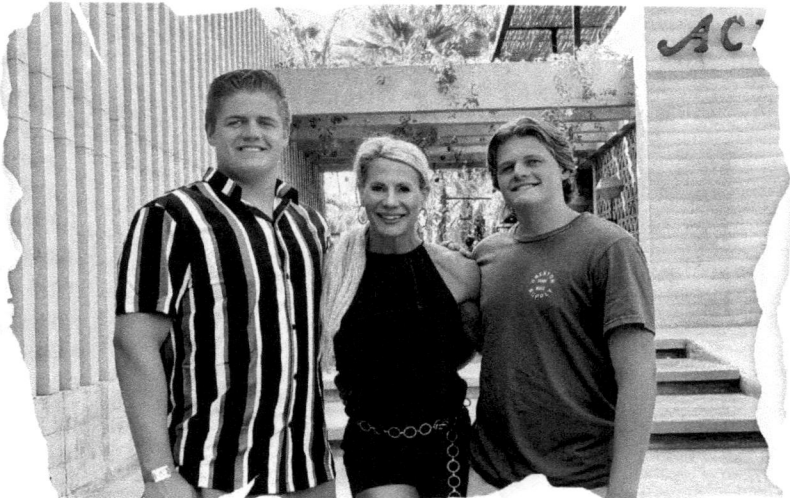

INTRODUCTION

Meet Whitney Jones—Unstoppable Energy in Human Form

When I was little, I didn't dream of being a princess or a doctor. I wanted to be a garbage truck. Not the driver, not the worker—the truck itself. Every day, I'd hear that rumble in the distance and my heart would leap. I would sprint to the backyard, climbing the wall to get the best view. The truck's arrival was electric. The clatter, the commotion, the sheer energy of it all—it wasn't just a moment; it was an event. For those few minutes, it didn't matter if my brothers and I had been fighting moments before. The garbage truck's arrival brought a shift, a spark of joy that could transform our entire day.

Looking back, it wasn't about the truck itself. What I truly admired was its power to ignite excitement and bring a sense of awe. Even as a child, I knew I wanted to have that same kind of impact. I wanted to stir something in people, to change the dynamic around them for the better. That desire has never left me. It's the core of who I am and the driving force behind the message and stories I now share with the world.

Growing up with two older brothers only added fuel to this fire. I was the youngest, the little sister, but they didn't treat me with kid gloves. There was no room for weakness in our house. If I wanted to keep up, I had to be tough. Sympathy wasn't part of the equation; grit was. If you got hurt, you threw some dirt on it and kept going. Those rough-and-tumble days didn't just toughen me up physically; they forged something deeper.

They instilled a resilience that would later become the foundation of what I call my "Win Broken" character.

That grit became my anchor when life's storms hit—and they hit hard. In a little over a year, my world was upended by a series of crushing blows. I took the leap to open a business, putting everything I owned on the line—my house, my car, my financial security. Just as I was navigating the pressures of entrepreneurship, I found myself lying beside my mom, my best friend, as she took her final breath after an aggressively fast and excruciating battle with cancer. Before I could even process that loss, I was blindsided by another—suddenly and unexpectedly becoming a single mom to my two little boys, just three and five years old. And as if that weren't enough, I uncovered that a trusted business partner had been stealing from the company, plunging it into debt and jeopardizing its future.

These moments could have crushed me. They could have turned me into a cautionary tale, another statistic, another train wreck. But I refused to let them define me. I chose resilience. I chose to rise. I chose to prove, not just to myself but to the world, that even when life leaves you broken, you can still find a way to win.

"Win Broken" isn't just a mantra; it's my story. It's about finding strength in the shards, about refusing to let circumstances dictate your worth. It's about making the conscious choice to turn pain into power, setbacks into stepping stones, and heartbreak into hope. That's the impact I've always wanted to have on the world, ever since those childhood days of chasing garbage trucks—to inspire, to excite, and to remind people that even in their brokenness, they have the power to win.

I WANT TO INSPIRE PEOPLE AND HAVE THEM SAY "WHITNEY, BECAUSE OF YOU I DIDN'T GIVE UP."

The Journey to Ms. Fitness Olympia

Hi, I'm Whitney Jones-mom, three-time Ms. Fitness Olympia, coach, business owner, unapologetic, donut, lover, and queen of doing what needs to be done when life says, "good luck with that." I'm also held together (quite literally) by a 12-piece metal cage in my neck, I've had 18 surgeries by the time of this writing, have broken almost every bone in my body and have enough determination to power a small country.

When people hear I'm a four-time World Champion, they assume my life must've been a straight shot to the top. Cue the laugh track. I wasn't some gymnastic prodigy tumbling my way to greatness as a kid. In fact, I didn't even know fitness competitions were a thing until I stumbled upon one in my early 30's. Up until that point, my athletic resume consisted of competing in high school and college sports and a few post-college endurance events. Nothing extraordinary.

So, how does someone go from "ordinary mom trying to stay fit" to becoming a world champion? The answer is grit—and a little bit of stubbornness. My first competition was a trainwreck. I forgot parts of my routine, tripped during a tumbling pass, and nearly fell off the stage. But you know what? I loved it. The adrenaline, the challenge, the opportunity to push myself—it was like nothing I'd ever experienced.

Fast-forward 7 years, and I was standing on the Olympia stage with a metal cage in my neck, a repaired ACL, and more setbacks than I could count. But I wasn't there despite my struggles—I was there *because* of them. They made me tougher, smarter, and more determined to win on my own terms.

Let me be clear about something: At the elite level of fitness competition, injuries aren't a matter of clumsiness or bad luck—they're an inevitable part of pushing the human body past what it's meant to do. When you're competing at the highest level in the world, testing the boundaries of human performance, injuries are a matter of "when," not "if." Just like professional football players, UFC fighters, or Olympic gymnasts, almost every top athlete in my sport faces injuries. We're not being reckless—we're pushing limits in pursuit of excellence. It's not about if you'll get injured—it's about how you handle it when you do. Do you let it stop you, or do you find a way to win broken? That's what defines a champion.

And for me, finding that way to win broken has always been driven by something bigger than titles. Above all else, my biggest motivation has always been my boys. Every time I step on stage, push through an injury, or face a new challenge, I think about them watching. I want them to see that their mom doesn't just talk about perseverance—she lives it. But it's grown beyond that. Through coaching and competing, I've realized that sharing our struggles honestly can create ripples of impact we never imagined. When one person stands up and says "I'm broken but still fighting," it gives others permission to do the same. That's why I'm here, showing you my scars, my setbacks, and my imperfect victories.

Why I Wrote This Book

Win Broken exists not because I have all the answers or a perfect life (spoiler: I don't). It's because I know what it feels like to be stuck—to want more but not know how to get there. Whether you're trying to get fit, build a business, find balance, or just make it through the day, this book is here to remind you of one thing: you're capable of more than you think.

This isn't a "rah-rah, you can do it" book filled with vague inspiration. It's a blueprint for tackling life head-on, even when the odds are stacked against you. I'll share my story—not because it's perfect, but because it's real. I'll give you the tools, strategies, and mindset shifts that have worked for me and my clients. And, of course, I'll throw in a little humor along the way. Because if we can't laugh through the chaos, what's the point?

So, grab your coffee (or popcorn) and settle in. Let's figure out how to win—broken pieces and all.

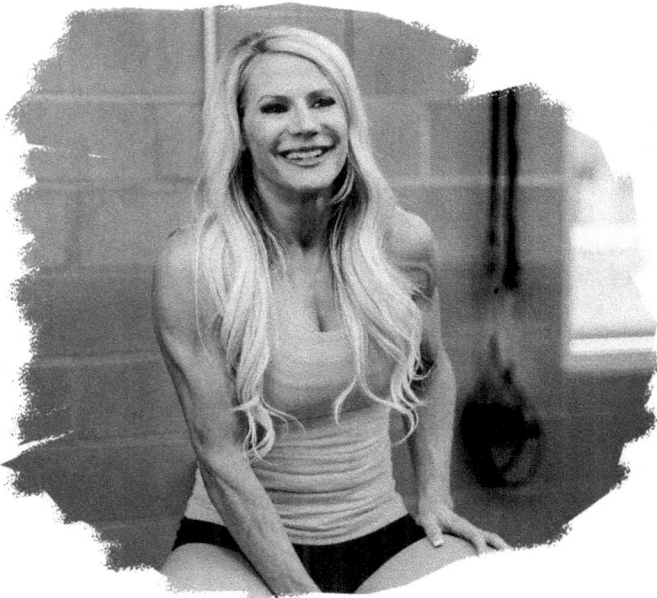

THE HIGH SCHOOL ATHLETE'S COMEBACK

Y ou never know when your story is going to change someone's life. In 2019, I got this message that hit me right in the heart from someone I'd never met. A high school football player—this incredible athlete with NFL dreams—had torn his ACL and completely shut down. We're talking full isolation mode: locked in his room, shutting out his friends, family, everyone. Nothing could pull him out of this dark place.

Until he watched Generation Iron 3.

Now, here's the wild part—this kid saw me talking about my injuries, my setbacks, my moments of thinking "this is it, game over." And something clicked. Here was someone who'd been broken (literally, in my case) and still found a way to win. Suddenly, his ACL tear wasn't a career-ender; it was just another chapter in his comeback story.

This kid went from "my life is over" to "watch me come back stronger" practically overnight. He attacked his rehab like it was his job. Double sessions, extra work, whatever it took. While his friends were hanging out after school, he was in physical therapy, rebuilding himself piece by piece. That's the thing about comebacks—they're not just about healing the injury; they're about rebuilding your spirit.

His mom told me later she had no idea what sparked the change—her son just woke up one day with this unstoppable fire to get back on the field. She said it was like watching a light switch back on. One day he was lost in the darkness, and the next, he was mapping out his comeback with the kind of determination that gives you chills.

Not only did he crush his recovery, but he landed that college scholarship he'd been dreaming of. Talk about a plot twist! The kid who thought his athletic career was over before it really began was now signing his letter of intent. Sometimes our biggest setbacks set us up for our greatest comebacks.

Here's what gets me: I was just sharing my story, my struggles, my battles. I had no idea it would help some kid in his darkest moment find his fight again. But that's the thing about being real about our broken moments—it gives other people permission to believe in their own comeback story. It shows them that being broken isn't the end; sometimes it's just the beginning.

That's why I share everything now—the wins, the losses, the moments of doubt, all of it. Because you never know who needs to hear exactly what you've been through to believe in what they can overcome.

Because sometimes all we need is to see someone else get back up to believe we can too.

Part 1: The Warrior Mindset

Turning Setbacks into Comebacks

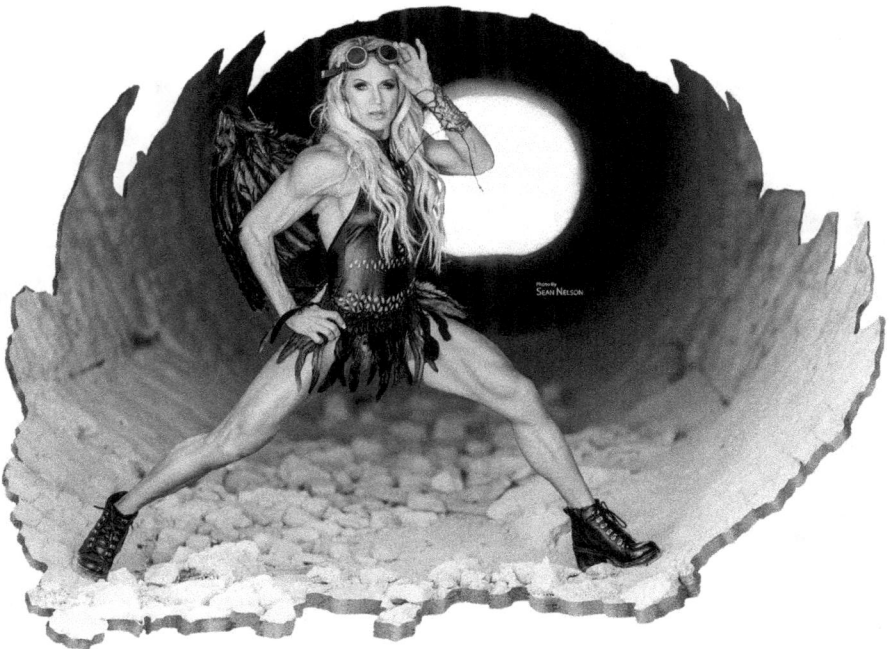

CHAPTER 1

Embracing the Hard Stuff

"YOU CAN'T CHEAT THE GRIND. IT KNOWS HOW MUCH YOU HAVE INVESTED. IT WON'T GIVE YOU ANYTHING YOU HAVEN'T WORKED FOR."
– *Whitney Jones*

There is a universal truth about life: it doesn't care about your plans. You can have the most perfectly curated vision board with glitter and motivational quotes, and life will still come barreling through like a toddler with a juice box—messy, unpredictable, and completely unbothered by your schedule.

I broke my neck—and didn't even realize it at first. I was practicing head spins, pushing myself to go faster and faster. Like any good athlete with questionable judgment, I went home and got my snowboard helmet, thinking that would help me spin even faster on the carpet.

Here's where the story takes a turn (pun intended). The helmet did make me spin faster—way faster than I should have been going. During my head spin variation, I pop off my head and flip into a splat landing on my back. But with the extra speed from the helmet and the carpet's traction, something went wrong. My neck slipped, and I crashed into my landing.

At first, I thought I'd just tweaked my shoulder again—it wasn't my first rodeo with shoulder injuries. Being the stubborn athlete I am, I went back later that same day to practice gainer flips into a push-up position. But something was off. My arm wasn't catching me like it should. I kept face-planting, and I knew I needed to call it a day.

A couple days later, I went to see my sports therapist for what I thought was another shoulder issue. When she pressed on the back of my neck, she found a pocket of fluid—a possible sign of a broken neck. She immediately stopped the session and told me I needed to see a neurosurgeon. I thought she was being dramatic. Spoiler alert: she wasn't.

She was so concerned that she called my friend Sally Williams to make sure I actually went to the doctor. Good thing too, because the diagnosis was clear: my neck was broken and I needed surgery. But here's where things got complicated—insurance wouldn't cover me, and the surgery cost $120,000. I ended up waiting weeks for approval, as I lost more and more function in my arm day by day.

In the end, they put me back together with a 12-piece metal cage, but that's a whole other story. The wild part? I still don't know exactly when I broke it—was it during the head spin, or did it happen during those gainer flips when I was already injured? Either way, it's a reminder that sometimes the most dangerous moments are when we think we're just pushing ourselves a little harder than usual.

Looking back, I probably should have listened to my body sooner. Maybe don't try this one at home.

Whitney's Totally Scientific Stages of Hard Stuff

1. **Denial**: *This can't be happening. Maybe I just injured my shoulder.*

2. **Drama**: *My life is OVER! Cancel everything!* (Cue dramatic music.)

3. **Acceptance-ish**: *Okay, this sucks. What's next?* (Usually said through a mouthful of yummy donut holes.)

4. **Action**: *Let's do this. Neck brace and all.* (Cue me attempting to work out without looking like a turtle flipped on its back.)

Here's what I learned: the hard stuff is where the magic happens. Sure, it's uncomfortable and annoying, and sometimes it makes you want to throw a tantrum (which I recommend, by the way—it's very therapeutic). But it's also where you grow. It's where you find out what you're made of.

Your Hard Stuff, Your Superpower

Look, I don't know what your version of the neck brace is. Maybe it's a bad breakup, a career setback, or the fact that your dog ate your favorite shoes. Whatever it is, here's my advice: embrace it. Scream into a pillow if you need to, but then figure out how you're going to rise. Because you can.

THE TROPHY IS EARNED IN THE HOURS THAT NO ONE IS WATCHING

Your Hardest Moments are Your Greatest Opportunities.

Life doesn't care about your plans—but you control how you respond. You've faced setbacks, moments of doubt, pain, and obstacles that felt impossible. Maybe you're experiencing one right now.

Here's the truth: those challenging moments—the neck-brace moments—hold the power to transform you.

At Empowering Legends, we turn your struggles into superpowers. We guide you through discomfort toward growth. It's not easy, but it's where the magic happens.

Join a community that doesn't just talk about resilience—we live it. Your legend isn't written in the spotlight; it's earned in the shadows, in those hours when no one is watching.

Are you ready to embrace your journey and discover what you're truly made of?

Take the next step. Your legend awaits.

EmpoweringLegends.com

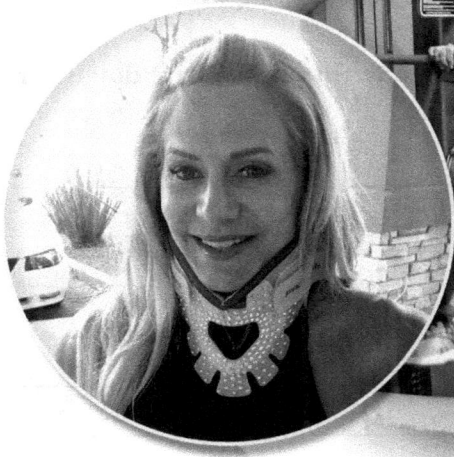

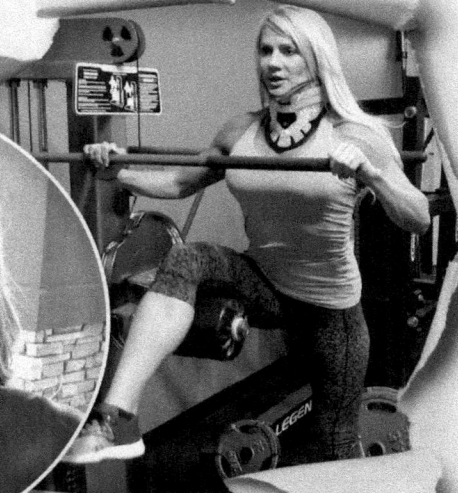

Lay in bed in a neck brace? I don't think so... time to add bling to the brace and hit the gym Whitney Style!

Your Turn:

Think about a tough time you've gone through. Write down three things it taught you.

_____

_____

_____

_____

_____

_____

_____

_____

_____

_____

_____

_____

Celebrate the fact that you survived it. Do a happy dance, treat yourself to a donut, or just say, "Dang, I'm a badass!" Because you are. (Write down what you celebrated and how it made you feel)

_____

_____

_____

_____

_____

_____

_____

_____

_____

_____

_____

_____

_____

_____

_____

_____

_____

_____

_____

_____

_____

CHAPTER 2

Fear as Your Superpower

"MENTAL TOUGHNESS IS BELIEVING WITHOUT A DOUBT, THAT WHATEVER HAPPENS, YOU GOT THIS." – *TIM GROVER*

Let's talk about fear. Not the casual "oh no, they're out of my favorite candy bar" kind of fear, but the real, heart-pounding, "what am I thinking?" kind of fear that makes you question all your life choices.

There was the time I went skydiving. Here's the thing: I'm terrified of heights. Like, sweaty-palms, racing-heart, can't-look-down terrified. But there I was at a bar with friends, and someone suggests, "Let's go skydiving tomorrow!" My mouth says "Yeah!" before my brain can process what's happening. You know that moment when your mouth writes a check your body isn't sure it wants to cash? That was me.

The next morning, reality hits. I'm standing there, about to jump out of a perfectly good airplane, wondering what life decisions led me to this moment. But here's where it gets interesting: in our group, I was the most scared but ended up being the most calm during the actual jump. Several people who talked a big game didn't even show up.

That day taught me something crucial about fear: it's not about being fearless—it's about being brave enough to say "watch me" when fear is screaming "you can't."

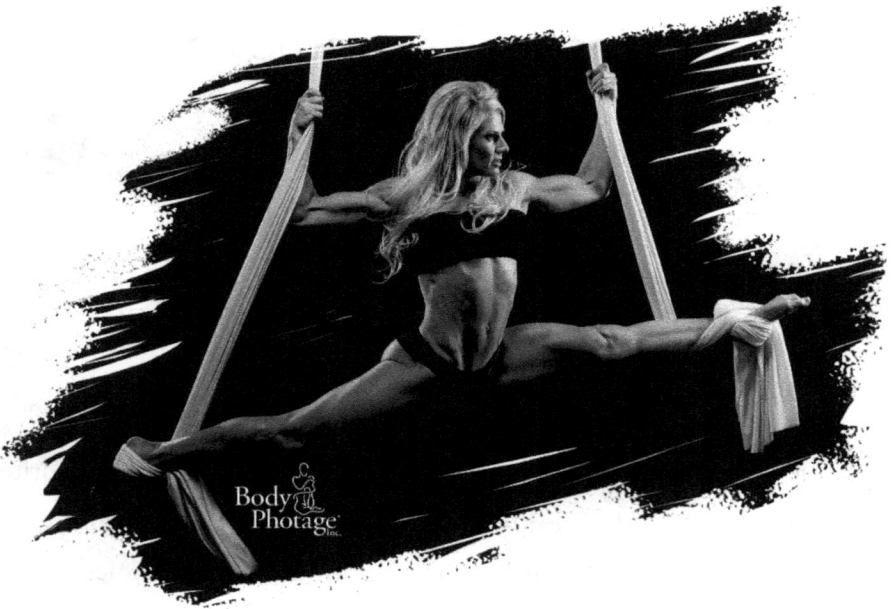

The Fun Side of Fear

Fear has been my co-pilot for most of my life. Whether it's stepping on stage, launching a new business, or back when I was trying to survive one of my kids' middle school science projects (seriously, why is there always glue everywhere?), fear is always there. And instead of running from it, I've learned to work with it. Sometimes I even laugh at it.

Take the time I decided to perform with a blown ACL. Every jump was like playing Russian roulette with my knee, and fear was screaming, "YOU CAN'T DO THIS!" But somewhere in that fear, I found the courage to say, "Watch me." And yes, I survived—and yes, I ate pizza after, because that's how champions celebrate.

How to Befriend Fear (Without Letting It Take Over Your Life)

1. **Name It**: Give your fear a funny name like "Captain Try Me." Whenever Captain Try Me shows up, say, "Oh hey, Cap. Fancy seeing you here. Let's do this thing anyway."

2. **Use It**: Fear is energy. Channel it. That skydiving fear? It became the confidence to try new moves in my routines. Because once you've jumped out of a plane, attempting a new flip doesn't seem quite so scary.

3. **Reward Yourself for Facing It**: Even if you just take one tiny step, celebrate it. Seriously. Fear hates it when you win, and I'm all about making fear mad.

The Domino Effect of Facing Fear

That skydiving experience did something amazing for my career. When fear would try to hold me back from trying new moves or skills that seemed impossible, I'd think, 'Hey, I was terrified of heights but still jumped out of a plane—I can handle this!' That perspective gave me the confidence to attempt things that seemed impossible. Whenever someone shows me an impressive new trick and asks "Can you do this?", my default answer has become "There's only one way to find out."

Your Turn: Let Fear Cheer You On

What's one thing fear is stopping you from doing? Write it down.

Now, imagine what could go right if you did it. Write that down, too.

Take one baby step toward it today—even if that step is just saying out loud, "I'm doing this."

Remember: the goal isn't to eliminate fear. It's to make fear your hype person. Let it energize you, motivate you, and push you toward things you never thought possible.

And if all else fails, just remember: you can either let fear write your story, or you can write it yourself—preferably while doing something that makes fear say, "Oh no she didn't!"

(Spoiler alert: Oh yes, she did!)

"DO IT BECAUSE THEY SAID YOU COULDN'T." –

Whitney Jones

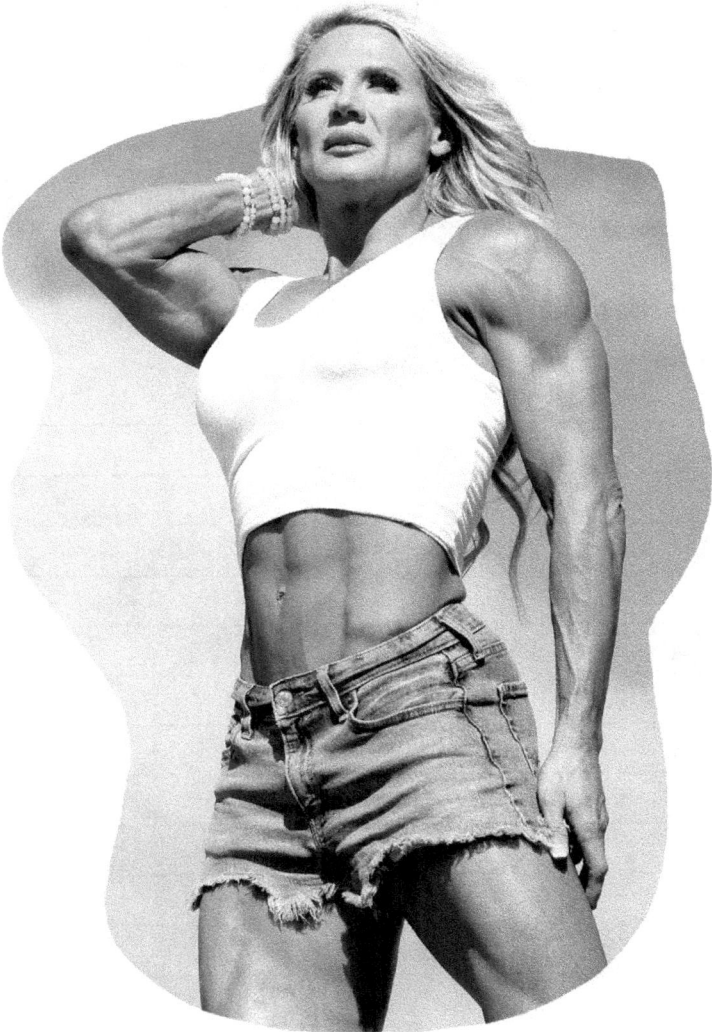

Your Turn:

What is the biggest fear that you've overcome?
What fears are you facing now?

_____
_____
_____
_____
_____
_____
_____
_____
_____
_____
_____
_____
_____

What could go right if you overcome this fear?

CHAPTER 3

Mindset Hacks Whitney Swears By

"SUCCESS IN LIFE COMES WHEN YOU SIMPLY REFUSE TO GIVE UP. WITH GOALS SO STRONG THAT OBSTACLES, FAILURE, AND LOSS ONLY ACT AS MOTIVATION." – *Dr. Merodie*

The power of mindset: Three days before the 2021 Ms. Fitness Olympia—the biggest competition of the year—I broke my leg. Most people would have withdrawn, but here's the thing about mindset: it's not about what happens to you, it's about how you choose to handle it.

I didn't tell anyone except my closest team members. No X-rays, no doctor visits, because I knew what they'd say. Instead, I looked at myself in the mirror and said, "What's done is done. We're not focusing on what we can't change. We're focusing on what we can do."

You want to know the truth about mindset? It's not some magical, woo-woo thing that only elite athletes or motivational speakers have mastered. It's messy, it's unpredictable, and sometimes it's just about convincing yourself to keep going even when your brain is screaming, "This is insane! You can't perform a two-minute routine with a broken leg!"

But here's what I did: I completely redesigned my routine—in my head. No practice runs (hello, broken leg!), no rehearsals. Just pure visualization and an unwavering belief that I could pull this off. And you know what? I won my third Ms. Fitness Olympia title that year.

Was it pretty? Maybe not. Was it perfect? Far from it. But it proved something I've always believed: your mind can push you past any limitation if you let it.

Hack #1: Play the "What's Next?" Game

When life hits you with a setback (or you know, a broken leg three days before the biggest competition of your life), it's easy to spiral. Your brain starts throwing a pity party, complete with sad balloons and that one playlist you only listen to when you're feeling sorry for yourself. Been there, done that.

But instead of getting stuck in the "Why me?" loop, I play a little game called "What's Next?" It's simple: instead of dwelling on what went wrong, I ask myself, "What can I do right now to move forward?" Sometimes the answer is big (like redesigning an entire routine), and sometimes it's small (like eating some chocolate and taking a deep breath). Either way, it keeps you moving.

"IT'S NOT WHO YOU THINK YOU ARE THAT HOLDS YOU BACK. IT'S WHO YOU THINK YOU'RE NOT." – *Whitney Jones*

Hack #2: Give Yourself a Pep Talk

Look, I get it—talking to yourself feels weird. But here's the thing: your brain is already talking to you 24/7. It's telling you stories about who you are, what you can do, and what's possible. So why not take control of the narrative?

When I was standing backstage at the Olympia, trying to ignore the throbbing in my leg, I told myself, "You've done hard things before, and you can do them again. This is just another challenge to overcome." It wasn't about lying to myself—it was about reminding my brain that I'm stronger than it thinks.

Hack #3: Make It Fun

If there's one thing I know for sure, it's that laughter is a superpower. Even in serious situations (like competing for a world title with a broken leg), finding moments of humor helps you push through. I remember glancing at my best friend and fellow fitness pro, Sally Williams, right before going on stage and whispering, "Aren't you going to tell me to go break a leg?" as I looked down at my bruised and swollen leg. Was it a terrible joke? Absolutely. Did it help calm my nerves? You bet.

Your Mindset To-Do List

This week, try one of these hacks:

1. When something goes wrong, ask yourself, "What's next?" (And if the answer is "eat a snack," that's valid.)

2. Give yourself a pep talk in the mirror. Start with, "You've got this, and Whitney says so."

3. Find one thing to laugh about every day. It doesn't matter if it's a meme, a blooper reel, or your own ridiculous attempt at making the best of a tough situation—just laugh.

Remember: your mindset is a muscle. The more you work on it, the stronger it gets. And like any muscle, it's going to get sore, tired, and occasionally make you want to throw in the towel. But if I can train my brain to push through a broken leg at the Olympia, then trust me—you can train yours to handle whatever challenges come your way.

Now, who's ready to work on those mindset gains? (And yes, snacks are allowed during training.)

Life will always test you—but your mindset determines your victory.

You've faced setbacks, doubt, pain, and obstacles that seemed impossible. But here's the secret: those moments are your greatest opportunities.

At Empowering Legends, we believe that true success happens when you refuse to give up. When you transform obstacles into motivation, your challenges become your superpower.

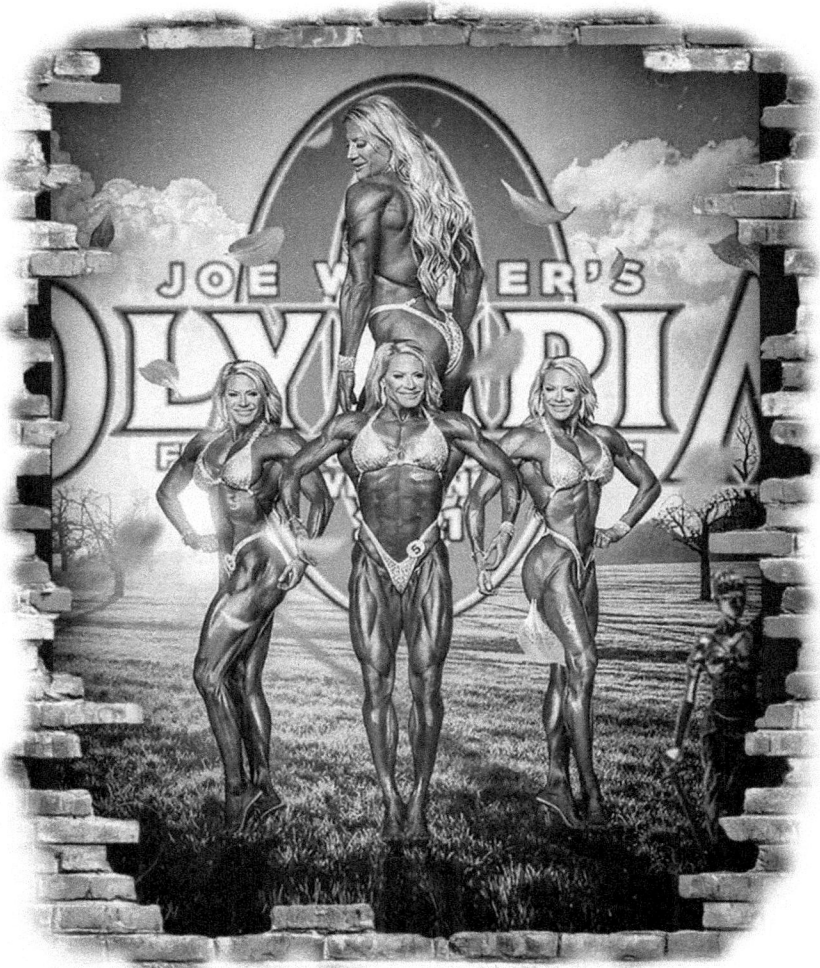

Join a community dedicated to building resilience and redefining limits. Your legend isn't written in the spotlight; it's forged in your unwavering determination to keep going, even when it feels impossible.

Are you ready to strengthen your mindset and claim your victory?

Take the next step. Your legend awaits.

EmpoweringLegends.com

YOUR TURN:

List any setbacks you are facing, and then write out what's next:

_____

_____

_____

_____

_____

_____

_____

_____

_____

_____

_____

_____

_____

_____

What have you laughed about recently?
(These will be fun to look back on)

_____

_____

_____

_____

_____

_____

_____

_____

_____

_____

_____

_____

_____

_____

_____

_____

_____

_____

_____

_____

CHAPTER 4

The Comeback Is Always Better Than the Setback

"STRENGTH DOES NOT COME FROM WINNING. YOUR STRUGGLES DEVELOP YOUR STRENGTHS. WHEN YOU GO THROUGH HARDSHIPS AND DE-CIDE NOT TO SURRENDER, THAT IS STRENGTH."
- *ARNOLD SCHWARZENEGGER*

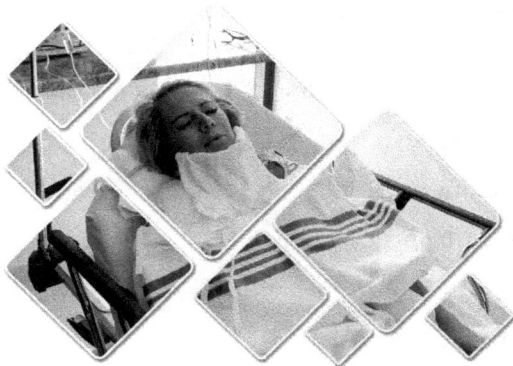

Nine months into recovery from neck surgery, where doctors literally put my neck back together with a 12-piece metal cage. My goal was clear—I was determined to make my comeback at the 2018 Arnold Classic. I counted down the days until the competition and made the very most of each and every one of them. I shared every step of my recovery journey on social media, from the small victories to the major milestones.

But not everyone believed in my comeback story. The skeptics were having a field day, claiming I was posting old videos and lying about my recovery. They said I'd never compete again.

And then—because apparently having a bionic neck wasn't enough of a challenge—I tore my ACL just four weeks before the 2018 Arnold Classic.

Now, let's break this down: I had very limited upper body strength because of the neck surgery, and suddenly I had only one functioning leg. Most people would call it quits. Heck, most people wouldn't have even started. But here's what I knew: this wasn't just about a competition anymore. This was about proving something to myself, and I was up to the challenge.

The Whitney Comeback Method

1. **Pause and Breathe**: First things first—stop panicking. I sat in my gym, tears streaming down my face just days after tearing my ACL, looking at all the skills I couldn't do anymore. Then I took a deep breath and asked myself, "Okay, what CAN I do?" (Bonus points if you can do this without swearing under your breath. I usually fail at that part.)

2. **Decide to Own It**: Instead of hiding my limitations, I decided to work with them. Couldn't do my usual routine? Fine. I'd create something new that played to my current strengths. When you can't change the situation, change your approach.

3. **Add a Little Flair**: If you're going to make a comeback, do it with style. When I tore my ACL, I redesigned my entire routine around what I could do with one leg and limited upper body strength. And guess what? I didn't just compete—I won my first world championship title: the 2018 Arnold Classic Ms. Fitness International. Style points for making my leg brace part of my costume. Arnold Schwarzenegger even said that he didn't realize I was wearing a brace, he thought my costume had added coolness.

When the Show REALLY Must Go On

Speaking of proving things to myself, allow me to tell you about the time I dislocated my shoulder during the 2023 Olympia. Not just a minor dislocation—I'm talking full shoulder separation, torn rotator cuff, AND a broken collarbone. Mid-routine. On the biggest stage in our sport. Broadcast live worldwide.

In that moment, I faced a brutal choice. The logical move was clear: walk off stage and head to the hospital. But that meant automatic disqualification - a DNF (Did Not Finish) which wasn't an option for me. With no qualified medical staff on-site for this kind of injury, I made what was probably a terrible decision. I went backstage, took a deep breath, and did something you should absolutely never try: I popped my own shoulder back into place. Then I walked back out to finish the show.

Why? Because my boys were watching, and I needed them to see that when you commit to something, you see it through—even when it feels impossible, even when it hurts, even when every logical part of your brain is screaming "STOP!" If there's a way forward, I'll find it. And in that moment, between the pain and the screaming logic, I found mine.

You want to talk about comebacks? These weren't just comebacks—these were "hold my protein shake and watch this" moments.

Real-Life Comeback Stories

Those victories made headlines, but let me tell you about some other comebacks that didn't make it into the movies (oh yeah, one actually did—catch it in Generation Iron 3).

Like the time my bikini broke during the Hawaii Pro in the middle of my Physique Judging Round. There I am, doing my model turns, when snap—wardrobe malfunction central. Did I run off stage? Nope. I adjusted, covered strategically, and kept going. Because that's what you do when life tries to literally expose you—you adapt and keep moving.

Or how about the time I completely blanked on my routine mid-performance when I was an amateur? For a second, I froze. But then I thought, "Well, standing here awkwardly isn't going to win anything." So, I improvised. I threw in a few extra dance moves, struck a pose, and acted like I planned it all along. The crowd loved it, and I learned something important: people don't remember the stumble—they remember how you recover.

Your Turn: Plan Your Comeback

The next time something goes wrong (because let's be real, it will), ask yourself: How can I recover with confidence? Practice your "comeback pose," whether it's a power stance, a goofy grin, or your best slow clap. And remember: the comeback is always better than the setback.

Whitney's Comeback Rules to Live By

1. **Redefine Success**: Sometimes winning doesn't look like what you originally planned. Be open to rewriting your definition of victory. (Sometimes victory means finishing a routine with only half your working parts, and that's okay!)

2. **Use the Doubters as Fuel**: Those social media skeptics? They became my rocket fuel. Nothing motivates quite like proving people wrong.

3. **Keep Your Sense of Humor**: That torn ACL gave me a limp, but I played it off as swagger. 'Nah, I'm not limping—just got a little extra swag these days.'

4. **Document the Journey**: Take pictures, write notes, record your progress. Trust me, looking back at where you started makes the

comeback even sweeter. (Plus, it makes for great social media content—just saying.)

"WORK HARD IN SILENCE, LET SUCCESS MAKE THE NOISE." – Frank Ocean

The Real Secret to Epic Comebacks

Here's the truth about comebacks: they're not about being perfect. They're about being persistent. They're about looking at a seemingly impossible situation and saying, "Watch me."

When I stepped onto that Arnold Classic stage—with my bionic neck and my busted knee—or when I finished that Olympia routine with my shoulder barely staying in its socket, I wasn't just competing. I was making a statement: You can't break what's already broken and I'm still standing.

So, what's your comeback going to be? Whatever it is, remember: if I can win a world championship with essentially one and a half functioning limbs, or finish the competition after DIY shoulder reconstruction, you can absolutely overcome whatever setback you're facing right now.

And hey, if all else fails, strike a pose and pretend you meant to do that. Works every time.

(Well, almost every time. Let's not talk about that one competition where I tried this and ended up doing an unplanned split. Thank goodness for stretchy costumes.)

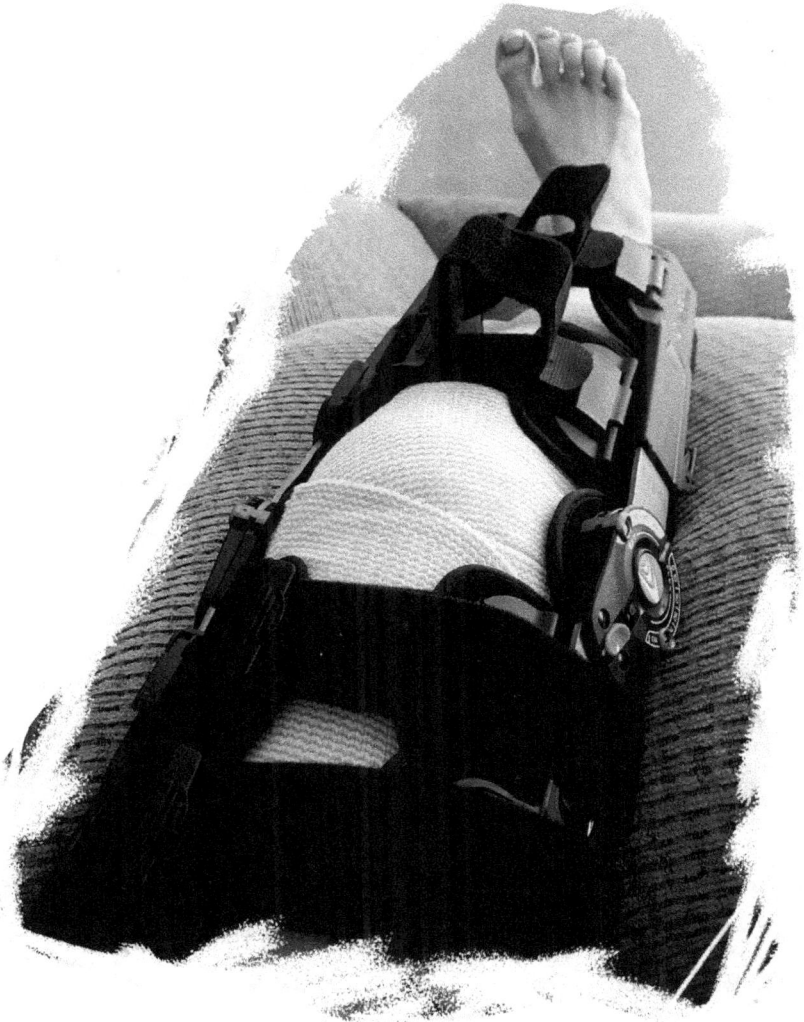

At home hours after surgery. Readjusting my goals since this injury wasn't part of my plan.

Your Turn:

What was your biggest setback in life?

_____

_____

_____

_____

_____

_____

_____

_____

_____

_____

_____

_____

_____

_____

What good came from this setback?

_____

_____

_____

_____

_____

_____

_____

_____

_____

_____

_____

_____

_____

_____

_____

_____

_____

_____

_____

_____

_____

_____

_____

Darren's Journey: Small Steps to Lasting Change

One of my earliest personal training clients, Darren Demayo, taught me something incredible about transformation—it's not just about hitting a goal, it's about creating a whole new way of life. When we first started working together, he was in the food and beverage industry, which is basically like trying to stick to your nutrition plan while working in a candy store. Talk about testing your willpower!

For about a year and a half, we worked together, building habits that could stand up to real-life challenges. That's the thing about lasting change—it has to work in your actual life, not just in some perfect bubble. And Darren's life was all about food and drinks; it was his passion, his career, his world. We couldn't change that (and honestly, we didn't want to), but we could figure out how to make health and career coexist.

Even after our training wrapped up due to financial changes, Darren had internalized something powerful: sustainable transformation isn't about temporary fixes or quick wins. It's about developing tools you can use for life. Like having a GPS for your health journey—when you get off track (because we all do), you know exactly how to redirect yourself back to where you want to be.

To this day, Darren occasionally checks in with updates that make me smile. His message is always the same: "Everything you taught me stuck with me. I'm not perfect—there are times when work events throw me off track—but I always hear your voice in my head about small steps leading to big things. When things start sliding, I know exactly how to pull it back."

What makes his story so powerful is how he's managed to blend his passion for the food industry with his commitment to wellness. It's not about choosing between your career and your health—it's about finding ways to make both work together. Sometimes that means saying yes to trying that new burger at work (because it's literally his job).

Darren's story perfectly demonstrates what I want everyone to take from this book: transformation isn't about achieving perfection—it's about developing the mindset and tools to keep going after setbacks. He learned that wellness isn't about never failing, but about having the confidence and know-how to get back on track when you do. Because let's be real—life isn't about avoiding all the loaded french fries. Sometimes it's about figuring out how to be the chef and still rock your fitness goals.

PART 2

Fearless Energy—Living with Passion and Humor

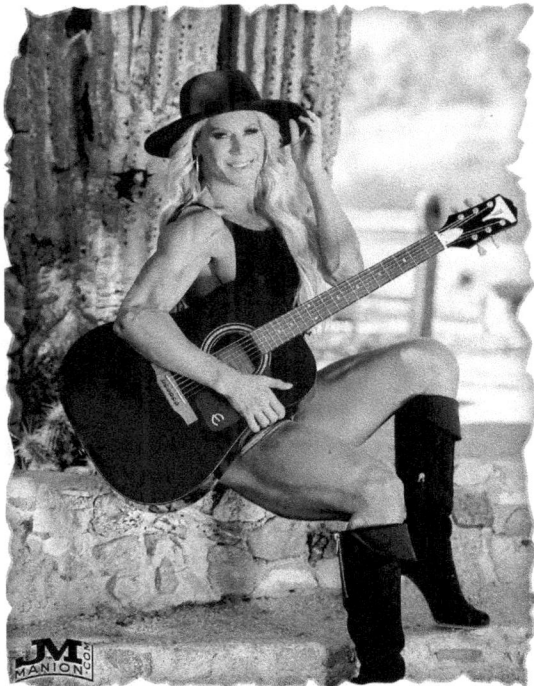

CHAPTER 5

Fitness, Fun, and Finding Your Flow

"EVERYTHING IS ENERGY. YOUR THOUGHTS
BEGIN IT, YOUR EMOTIONS AMPLIFY IT, AND
YOUR ACTIONS INCREASE ITS MOMENTUM."
- Whitney Jones

Here's a little-known fact: fitness doesn't have to feel like punishment. Shocking, right? Somewhere along the way, people decided that exercise had to be this grueling, joyless task where you sweat out every bad decision you've ever made. But guess what? They're wrong. Fitness can be fun—if you let it.

Let me prove it to you. Last week, I convinced a group of friends to try building human pyramids... in plank position. Picture this: grown adults stacking themselves like Jenga blocks, trying to hold perfect planks while laughing so hard they're shaking. Did we fall? Absolutely. Did we get an incredible core workout? You bet. Did someone's face end up in someone else's armpit? I plead the fifth.

Step 1: Redefine What "Fitness" Looks Like

Newsflash: fitness doesn't have to mean hours at the gym staring at yourself in those weirdly unflattering mirrors. (Seriously, why are they so unflattering?) Sometimes it's creating synchronized pushup combos with friends like we're auditioning for a fitness version of So You Think You Can Dance. Or it's attempting toe touches over rolling tires coming at you—because why not add an element of danger to your fitness routine?

For me, fitness is my happy place. It's where I go to clear my head, recharge my energy, and—let's be honest—burn off the snacks I ate the night before. But it's also where I have the most fun. There's nothing better than trying a new workout and realizing, "Hey, I actually like this!"

Step 2: Make It Ridiculously Fun

Remember when you were a kid, and "exercise" meant running around outside until the streetlights came on? Yeah, let's bring that energy back.

Here are some of my favorite ways to make fitness fun:

1. **Create Ridiculous Challenges**: My friends and I are constantly inventing new "stupid human tricks." The outtakes are always better than the actual workout. Trust me, nothing builds abs like laughing at yourself trying to do anything synchronized with a friend.

2. **Film the Fun**: Record your fitness adventures. Not because you

need to go viral, but because watching yourself attempt a back-flip off a wall (with proper safety measures, of course) is pure entertainment. Plus, you get some great blackmail material on your workout buddies.

3. **Make Everything a Game**: Who can hold a plank the longest while telling dad jokes? How many sit-ups can you do while your friend tries to make you laugh? The possibilities are endless.

Step 3: Keep It Simple

If you're just starting out, don't overcomplicate it. You don't need fancy equipment or a five-year plan. Start with what you've got: your body, a pair of sneakers, and maybe a decent playlist (When legit beats drop, they can be surprisingly motivating).

Whitney's Guide to Fun Fitness Fails

Here are some of my favorite fitness "experiments":

- The time we tried to create a human pyramid in plank position and ended up looking more like a collapsed card house.

- The synchronized pushup routine that turned into an impromptu face-plant competition.

- The "let's see who can jump over these rolling tires" challenge that taught us all about reflexes (and humility).

But here's the thing: these "fails" are actually wins. Because we're moving, we're laughing, and we're creating memories. Plus, my abs always get the best workout from laughing at our attempts.

"RULE YOUR MIND OR IT WILL RULE YOU."
- Horace

Making Friends with Fitness

Truth bomb: everything's more fun with friends. Here's why:

1. **Accountability with a Side of Fun**: Your workout buddy will show up, if only to watch you attempt that new move you've been bragging about.

2. **Creative Energy**: Two (or more) minds are better than one when inventing ridiculous workout challenges.

3. **Built-in Entertainment**: Someone will inevitably do something hilarious, and boom—instant core workout from laughing.

Your Turn: Make Fitness Fun

This week, try one new way to move your body. It doesn't matter if it's dancing, hiking, or attempting to teach your dog how to do squats (good luck). The goal is to find something that makes you smile—and maybe sweat a little.

Bonus: Whitney's Favorite Workout Games

1. 1 Minute Challenge: Count the number of push-ups, pull-ups, or sit-ups while telling jokes. Last one to break from laughing wins.

2. **Dance Break Burpees**: Every time a new song starts, drop and do five burpees. Make them as dramatic as possible.

3. **The Superhero Circuit**: Create exercises based on superhero moves. Points for creativity and sound effects. Examples: Spider-man Crawls or Ball Slams that mimic Hulk Smashes.

Remember: The best workout is the one you'll actually do. And you're more likely to do it if you're having fun. So stop taking it all so seriously. Get out there, try something new, maybe fall on your face a few times (safely, please), and remember that laughter burns calories too.

Just maybe avoid filming the human pyramid attempts. Or do film them, but know they might end up as evidence of what not to do in a future fitness safety video. Your choice.

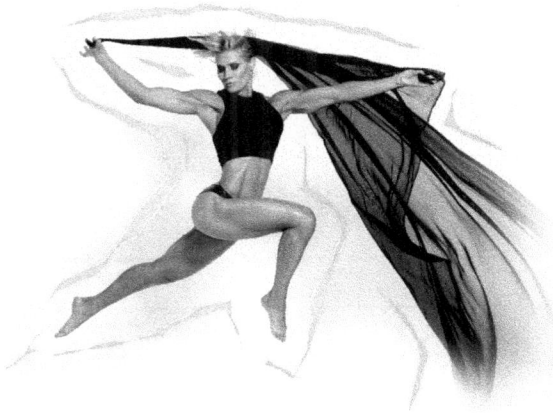

YOUR TURN:

What activities really light you up?

_____

_____

_____

_____

_____

_____

_____

_____

_____

_____

_____

_____

_____

_____

What's something silly you are going to try? (Safely)

CHAPTER 6

Balance, Not Perfection

"LIFE IS LIKE RIDING A BICYCLE. TO KEEP YOUR BALANCE YOU MUST KEEP MOVING." - *Einstein*

Raise your hand if you've ever made a perfectly scheduled day... and then life looked at your planner and said "That's cute." (Don't worry, I can't see you, but I know your hand is up.)

Here's the thing about balance: it's less like a perfect scale and more like juggling while riding a unicycle on a tightrope. During a hurricane. With your eyes closed. While someone keeps throwing random objects at you yelling "Here, just add this to the mix!"

Picture this: It's competition prep, just weeks from a major show. My day is perfectly planned—training, meals, business meetings—all color-coded in my calendar like I'm some kind of organization super-hero. Then boom—the school nurse calls. One kid's sick. My gym's alarm system is having a meltdown. Three clients need their sessions covered because we're short-staffed. And somehow I agreed to a last-minute live podcast interview. My carefully planned routine practice? Yeah, that's not happening today.

The H2G2 Philosophy (aka The Game-Changer)

This is where my favorite mantra comes in: You don't HAVE to, you GET to. I learned this the hard way, and now it's plastered all over my house—bathroom mirrors, kid's rooms, probably somewhere in the garage (though I can't confirm because, well, have you seen my garage?).

Instead of thinking:

- "I have to pick up my sick kid" → "I get to be there for my kid"

- "I have to cover these classes" → "I get to help my business thrive"

- "I have to adjust my training schedule" → "I get to prove how adaptable I am"

See what I did there? Same situations, totally different energy.

"DON'T CONFUSE YOUR PATH WITH YOUR DESTINATION. JUST BECAUSE IT'S STORMY NOW DOESN'T MEAN YOU AREN'T HEADED FOR SUNSHINE" - Trent Shelton

The Reality Check

Let's get real for a second: being a single mom, running multiple businesses, and training for the Olympia isn't exactly a recipe for perfect balance. Some days it looks less like balance and more like that time I tried to carry all my grocery bags in one trip (because two trips are for quitters, am I right?).

But here's what I've learned: Balance isn't about doing everything perfectly—it's about juggling what matters without dropping yourself in the process.

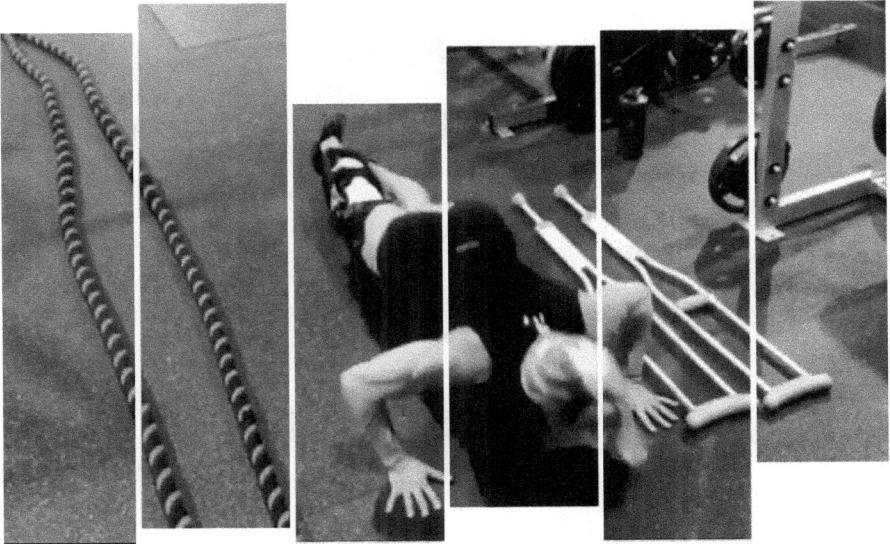

Back in the gym 48 hours post ACL surgery

Whitney's Not-So-Perfect Balance Blueprint

1. Plan Like a Boss, Pivot Like a Ninja:

- Have a schedule? Awesome.

- Ready to throw that schedule out the window when life happens? Even better.

- Keep your sense of humor when everything goes sideways? Now you're speaking my language.

2. **Focus on the Big Picture**:

- One missed workout won't kill your progress

- One imperfect meal won't ruin your diet

- One day of chaos won't derail your life

- Unless that chaos involves teaching your teenagers to drive—then all bets are off

3. **Listen to Your Body (and Your Schedule)**:

- Sometimes your body needs rest

- Sometimes your business needs attention

- Sometimes your kids need you

- Sometimes you need snacks (this is non-negotiable)

The Art of the Pivot

Remember that competition prep day I mentioned? Here's how it actually went down:

- Morning: Kid sick → School pickup → Work from home while playing nurse

- Mid-Morning: Call to fix the alarm issues and get clients covered for staff that's out

- Afternoon: Jumped on the unexpected podcast interview— unprepared but nailed it

- Evening: Modified routine practice in my living room while supervising homework

- Night: Collapse on couch, eat snacks, remind myself that **I get to** do all of this

Was it perfect? Nope. Did it work? Absolutely. Because perfect balance is a myth, but workable chaos? That's my specialty.

Real Talk: The Single Mom Superhero Strategy

Being a single mom while chasing massive goals taught me something: you can have it all, just not all at the same time, and definitely not all perfectly. And that's okay. Some days you're crushing it at work while the laundry piles up. Other days you're Mom of the Year while your email inbox blows up. The key is knowing that tomorrow's another day to readjust the juggling act.

51

The Permission Slip You Didn't Know You Needed

Here's your official permission (from someone who's mastered the art of beautiful disaster):

- It's okay if your balance looks different each day

- It's okay if some balls drop (just not the important ones, like children)

- It's okay to laugh when things go sideways

- It's absolutely okay to celebrate small wins with snacks

Your Turn: Finding Your Balance

This week, try this:

1. Write down everything you "have to" do

2. Change each one to "get to"

3. Notice how different it feels

4. Adjust as life throws curveballs (and it will)

5. Celebrate surviving with your favorite snack (sensing a theme here?)

Remember: Life is messy, schedules are guidelines, and sometimes the most balanced thing you can do is accept the chaos and keep moving forward—preferably with snacks and a sense of humor.

Because at the end of the day, you don't HAVE to do any of this. You GET to. And that perspective makes all the difference between surviving and thriving in the beautiful chaos of life.

Just maybe don't try the human pyramid in plank position on the days you're already struggling with balance. Trust me on this one.

Find your balance in the chaos—keep moving forward with **EmpoweringLegends.com**

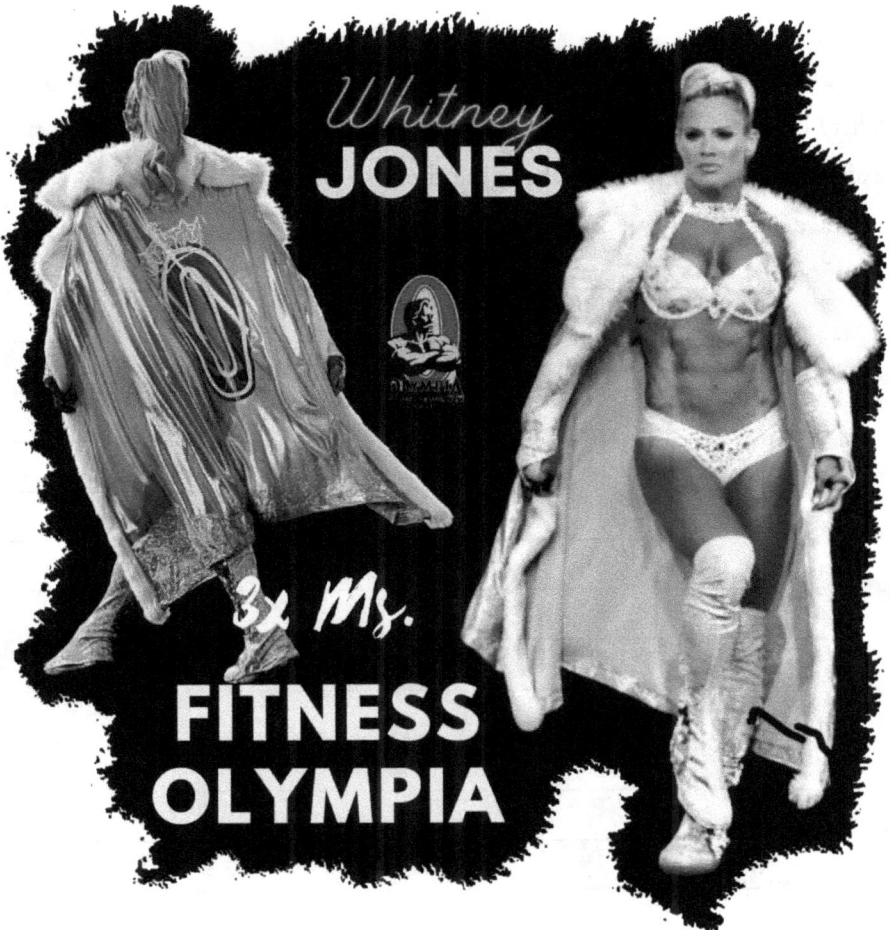

Your Turn:

Write out things you **HAVE TO DO** today or this week that you're not excited about and practice changing them to **GET TO DO**:

Have To: _____

Get To: _____

_____

Have To: _____

Get To: _____

_____

Have To: _____

Get To: _____

_____

Have To: _____

Get To: _____

_____

Have To: _____

Get To: _____

_____

Have To: _____

Get To: _____

_____

Have To: _____

Get To: _____

_____

Have To: _____

Get To: _____

_____

Have To: _____

Get To: _____

_____

Have To: _____

Get To: _____

_____

Have To: _____

Get To: _____

_____

Have To: _____

Get To: _____

_____

Have To: _____

Get To: _____

_____

Have To: _____

Get To: _____

_____

CHAPTER 7

Laughing Through the Chaos

"I DEFINE MY OWN LIFE. I DON'T LET PEOPLE WRITE MY SCRIPT." - Oprah Winfrey

Here's something they don't tell you about life: it's going to get messy. And sometimes, in the most serious moments, you're going to get the uncontrollable giggles. Like that time I had an important meeting with the Diamondbacks, and suddenly got hiccups. Not just any hiccups—the kind that make you laugh, which makes the hiccups worse, which makes you laugh harder.

My boss kept saying "Stop!" which is exactly the wrong thing to say to someone fighting both hiccups and inappropriate laughter. It's like telling someone "don't think about pink elephants." Guess what they're going to think about?

The Art of Recovering from Awkward Moments

Speaking of bosses and mortifying moments, I literally spit coffee in my boss's face. (Yes, the same boss from the hiccup fiasco.). Picture this. Important meeting, someone says something funny right as I take a sip of coffee, and instead of keeping it cool, I turn and... projectile coffee, right in the boss's face.

There's a moment after something like that happens where time seems to stand still, and you have two choices:

1. Die of embarrassment on the spot

2. Own it and find the humor

I chose option 2. Because really, what else can you do when you've just turned your boss into an unwilling participant in a coffee shower?

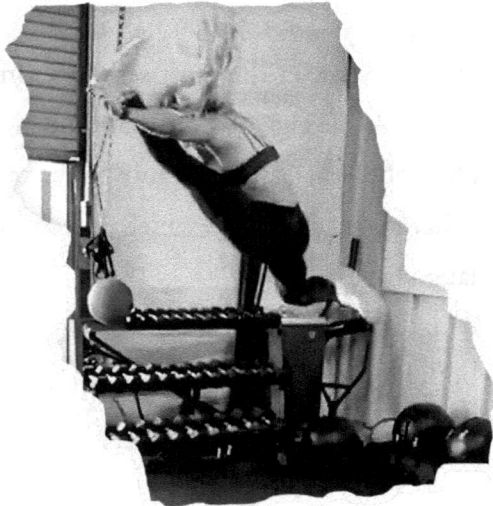

Shin to the face is never fun, especially when it's your own!

Whitney's Chaos Survival Kit

1. **Laugh First**: When something goes wrong, find the humor in it. Trust me, it's there—even if you have to dig a little.

2. **Own Your Moments**: Like that time we were celebrating a business win, and as we jumped for joy, I split my pants. Did I run away in shame? Nope. I struck a pose and said, "And that's why we always wear good underwear, folks!"

3. **Make It a Story**: Years from now, nobody's going to remember the perfect presentations or flawless meetings. They'll remember the time you had a laughing fit during an important call and snorted so loud it scared the IT guy.

Real-Life Examples of Chaos Management

Let's talk about church giggles. You know those moments—when you absolutely cannot laugh, which makes everything 100 times funnier? I'm the worst with these. During presentations, important meetings, quiet moments in church... my brain picks these times to remember something hilarious, and it's all downhill from there.

It's like my sense of humor has exactly zero respect for appropriate timing. But here's what I've learned: sometimes these simple moments of inappropriate joy are exactly what we need to break tension and remind us not to take life too seriously. Shake it off like a wet dog.

The Recovery Protocol

When you find yourself in one of these situations (and you will), here's what to do:

1. **Acknowledge the Moment**: There's no use pretending that coffee didn't just come out your nose.

2. **Find the Humor**: If people are going to remember this moment anyway, give them something good to remember.

3. **Keep It Moving**: Like that time I raced a valet in Scottsdale (bad idea), tripped, ripped my jeans, broke my heel, and ended up bloody. Did I go home? Nope! I rocked that "just survived a minor disaster" look all night. One shoe, ripped jeans, battle wounds and all.

The Power of the Recovery Dance

Sometimes, the best way to handle chaos is to quite literally dance through it. I once tried to bust out a back spin at a bar (wearing white, because apparently I make great decisions). Did I end up looking like I'd just mopped the dance floor? Yes. Did I turn it into an impromptu dance party? Also yes.

Your Turn: Find the Funny

This week, when life gets chaotic, stop and ask yourself, "What's funny about this?" If nothing comes to mind, just picture me in an important meeting with the hiccups, trying desperately not to laugh while my boss gets increasingly frustrated. See? You're smiling already.

Whitney's Rules for Chaos Navigation

1. **The Laugh Rule**: If you can laugh about it later, you might as well laugh about it now.

2. **The Story Rule**: If it's going to make a great story, it's worth the embarrassment.

3. **The Recovery Rule**: It's not about avoiding the chaos—it's about how fabulously you handle it.

Remember: Life is going to throw you curveballs. Sometimes those curveballs will be hiccups in important meetings. Sometimes they'll be coffee in your boss's face. And sometimes they'll be wardrobe malfunctions that test your ability to improvise.

The key isn't to avoid these moments—it's to embrace them, laugh through them, and maybe keep a spare pair of pants in your car. Just in case.

Because at the end of the day, the best stories never start with "So everything went exactly as planned..."

YOUR TURN:

Jot down some of your most embarrassing moments:

_____

_____

_____

_____

_____

_____

_____

_____

_____

_____

_____

_____

If these situations happened now, how would you handle them?

_____

_____

_____

_____

_____

_____

_____

_____

_____

_____

_____

_____

_____

_____

_____

_____

_____

_____

_____

_____

_____

_____

_____

_____

_____

Pat's Total Life Transformation

P at's story represents the kind of holistic change that happens when someone fully commits to their health journey. In his mid-50s, Pat signed up for our program looking physically unwell and lacking energy. What makes his transformation remarkable wasn't just the physical changes - it was watching his entire demeanor and approach to life evolve.

The turning point came when we asked him to take progress photos. While initially embarrassing, seeing those unflattering photos created a powerful moment of clarity. Pat realized just how far things had gotten and made a full commitment to change.

He approached the program with dedication but also grace for himself. Rather than trying to be perfect with his nutrition, he focused on making consistently better choices. Those small daily improvements began adding up. He established a morning routine that included hiking, giving himself time for mental reflection and recharging.

Within just three months, the changes were dramatic. Beyond losing weight and getting off various medications, Pat's confidence soared. His natural humor and easy-going personality, which had been muted by insecurity, came alive. He began confidently engaging with others and bringing his authentic self to every interaction.

Today, Pat is taking on physical challenges that would have seemed impossible a year ago - from Grand Canyon hikes to Spartan Races. He has maintained his great results by shifting his focus from pure weight loss to performance-based goals. This keeps him more consistent with healthy eating and regular activity, proving that sustainable transformation happens when we move beyond the scale to find deeper motivation.

His journey shows that it's never too late to start, and that true fitness transformation reaches far beyond physical changes to impact every aspect of life.

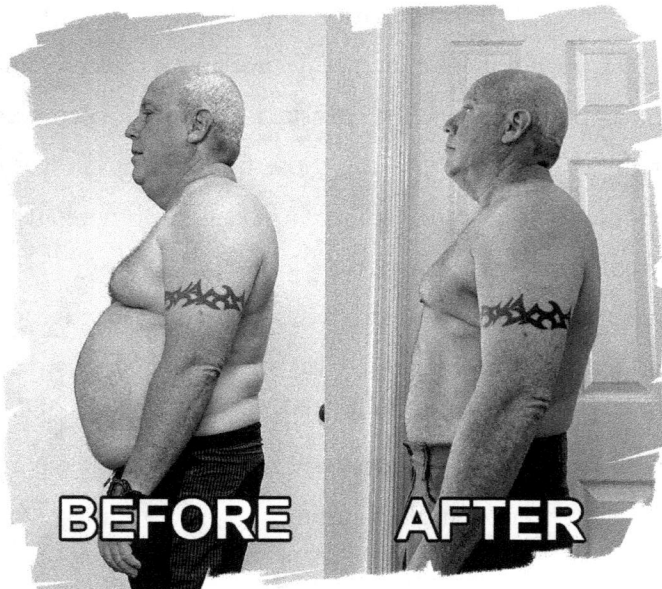

BEFORE   AFTER

PART 3

Rise with Whitney—Your Coach for All Life's Battles

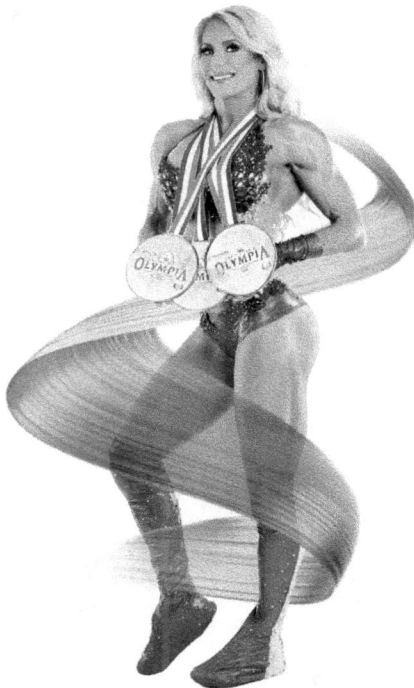

CHAPTER 8

Why I Coach

"FOCUS ON THE GOAL, NOT THE OBSTACLE." -
Whitney Jones

I love coaching. It's not just about helping people lose weight or hit personal records (though, trust me, watching someone crush a deadlift never gets old—it's like being a proud mama bear, except with more chalk and probably some questionable gym music in the background).

It's about being part of someone's transformation—physically, mentally, and emotionally. It's about watching someone go from "I can't" to "Watch me do this thing I swore was impossible while making it look ridiculously good." There's nothing like it.

The First Client Who Changed Everything

When I started coaching, I wasn't thinking about building a business or winning awards. I was just helping a friend who was doing the whole "juggling a million things while running on fumes" routine. You know the one—where coffee is basically a food group and dry shampoo is your best friend?

She told me, "I don't even know where to start." So, we started small. A 10-minute walk. Swapping soda for water. Sleeping an extra hour at night (which, let's be real, is like finding a unicorn for most busy people).

A few months in, she told me something I'll never forget: "You didn't just help me lose weight—you helped me find myself again." That's when I realized: coaching isn't just about fitness. It's about helping people rediscover their power, even if they're currently hiding it under a pile of laundry and self-doubt.

>"HARD DAYS ARE THE BEST BECAUSE THAT'S WHEN CHAMPIONS ARE MADE." - *Gabby Douglas*

Why I'm Obsessed with Progress

Here's a little secret: I'm not obsessed with perfection. I'm obsessed with progress. Perfection is boring, and let's be honest, it's about as realistic as a third-grader's dream of becoming a professional unicorn trainer.

Progress, though? That's where the magic happens. Every step forward is a win, whether it's:

- Lifting five more pounds

- Drinking more water

- Just showing up when your bed was staging a very convincing protest

- Finally nailing that one acrobatic skill you've been practicing (without face-planting)

Lessons Coaching Has Taught Me

1. **Everyone Has a Story**:
   Every client brings their own struggles, strengths, and goals. Some want to climb mountains, others just want to be able to chase their toddler without needing a nap immediately after. Both are equally valid goals, and both probably require snacks.

2. **Small Wins Add Up**:
   Big transformations don't happen overnight. They happen one small win at a time, kind of like building a LEGO castle. Except instead of losing pieces under the couch, you're building habits that last.

3. **It's Never Too Late**:
   I've coached people in their 40s, their 60s, even their 80s. The human body is incredible, and it's never too late to move in new ways. Though maybe we skip the backflips for the octogenarians.

The Real Coaching Moments

Some of my favorite coaching moments aren't the massive transformations—they're the little victories that probably look ridiculous to anyone watching:

- The client who was terrified of jumping rope and ended up mastering double-unders (after whipping herself in the shins approximately 847 times)

- The woman who thought she couldn't do push-ups and now drops into them randomly at social events (I may have created a monster)

- The guy who was so excited about his first pull-up, he did his victory celebration while still hanging from the bar (which, technically, counts as extra training)

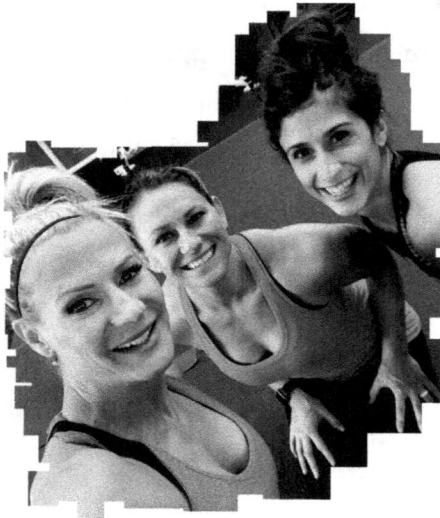

Why Every Session Is an Adventure

When you're a coach, you never know what each day will bring. One minute you're demonstrating proper squat form, the next you're trying to convince someone that no, they cannot work out while eating a burrito. (I mean, technically you can. But should you?)

Sometimes you're a:

- Fitness coach

- Life coach

- Therapist

- Professional cheerleader

- Snack consultant

- Professional face-plant preventer

And sometimes you're all of these things within the same five minutes.

Exercise: Your Coaching Reflection

Even if you're not a coach, you have the power to inspire and support others. Think about someone in your life who could use a few words of encouragement. How can you show up for them this week?

Write down one thing you can do to help them move forward. Maybe it's:

- A workout buddy session

- A motivational text

- A surprise healthy snack delivery

- Just being there to spot them (literally or figuratively)

Remember: Sometimes the best coaching happens when you're not trying to coach at all. Sometimes it's just about being there, believing in someone, and occasionally reminding them that yes, form matters more than how many likes their gym selfie gets.

Because at the end of the day, coaching isn't just about sets and reps—it's about helping people become the strongest version of themselves, inside and out.

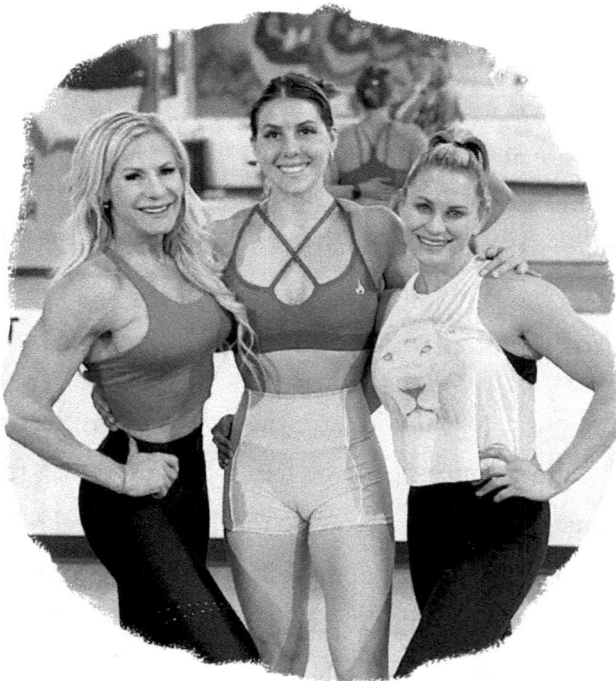

Your Turn:

How has a coach helped you achieve more?

_____

_____

_____

_____

_____

_____

_____

_____

_____

_____

_____

_____

_____

_____

_____

_____

How have you coached someone which helped them?

_____

_____

_____

_____

_____

_____

_____

_____

_____

_____

_____

_____

_____

_____

_____

_____

_____

_____

_____

_____

_____

_____

_____

_____

CHAPTER 9

The Team Mentality

"MOTIVATION IS WHAT GETS YOU STARTED. HABIT IS WHAT KEEPS YOU GOING!" – Jim Ryun

You know what's better than chasing your dreams? Chasing them with a team of people who've got your back—and maybe a few who are willing to spot you when you're attempting questionable workout moves that seemed like a good idea at the time.

A good team is like a family you choose—they cheer for you, challenge you, and occasionally call you out when you're being a little too stubborn (not that I'd know anything about that... okay, fine, I totally would).

There's Room at the Top (No, Really)

Here's something I live by: success isn't a limited-time offer with only a few spots available. There's room for everyone at the top—and it's actually way more fun up there when you bring others with you.

Think about it: What's the point of achieving something amazing if you're standing there alone, doing a victory dance with no one to join in? (And trust me, my victory dances need witnesses. They're both spectacular and slightly embarrassing.)

The Power of Community

One of the best things about running a gym is the community we've built. It's not just a place to work out—it's where people come to feel supported, challenged, and occasionally witness me demonstrate what not to do during a new move. I've seen:

- Friendships blossom

- Milestones celebrated

- Dance-offs spontaneously erupt (okay, I usually start those)

- People discover strengths they never knew they had

- And yes, sometimes people fall down... but they never fall alone

The Group Hug That Celebrated the Personal Win

Speaking of celebrations—there was this time when a client nailed their goal box jump for the first time, after months of building up confidence for her to attempt without failing. The entire gym erupted in cheers, before I knew it, we had a spontaneous group hug happening. Pretty sure it's the most wholesome thing that's ever happened in a weight room. Though maybe not the most hygienic, considering we were all pretty sweaty. (Note to self: maybe keep some extra deodorant in the Personal Win celebration kit.)

Building Your Dream Team

Your team doesn't have to be big—it just has to be full of people who:

- Believe in you

- Make you laugh

- Want to see you win

- Will tell you when your form is off (in life and in lifts)

- Know your coffee or tea order

- Understand that sometimes "just one more rep" means "please save me from myself"

The Real Secret of Teamwork

You know what happens when you celebrate others' successes? They celebrate yours too. It's like starting a chain reaction of awesome. When you empower others, that energy comes back to you—usually with bonus high-fives and maybe some party poppers if you're lucky.

Think of it this way: if you help someone else reach their goals, you've basically got a built-in celebration buddy for when you reach yours. It's like creating your own personal cheer squad, one supported person at a time.

Join a community that celebrates your wins, lifts you through challenges, and empowers your legend—start today at **EmpoweringLegends.com**.

The Final Rep

Remember: no one ever reached the top of the mountain alone. Even if it looks like they did, I guarantee there was a team of people behind them, probably holding snacks and extra water bottles.

So build your team. Celebrate their wins like they're your own. Create the kind of energy that makes people want to join in. And never doubt the power of a good group victory dance—even if your coordination is questionable. (Speaking from personal experience here.)

Because at the end of the day, the best teams aren't just about achieving goals—they're about making the journey so fun that you almost forget how hard you're working.

Almost. (Let's be real, you'll definitely feel those squats tomorrow.)

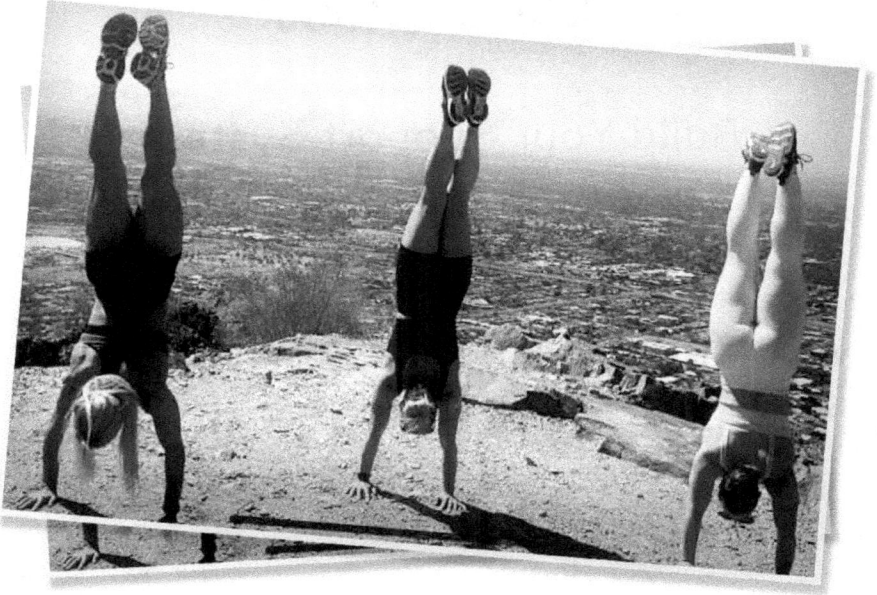

Handstand Fun

Your Turn:

Build Your Support System:

Who is your Dream Team? (Strong, Supportive, Inspiring)
Identify Them:

_____

_____

_____

_____

_____

Who can you show more support to?

_____

_____

_____

_____

_____

What do you need more support with?

_____

_____

_____

_____

_____

_____

_____

_____

_____

_____

How will you make that happen? What action are you taking?

_____

_____

_____

_____

_____

_____

_____

_____

_____

_____

_____

CHAPTER 10

Your Roadmap to Success

"OBSTACLES DO NOT BLOCK THE PATH, THEY ARE THE PATH." Zen Proverb

Goals without a plan are just wishes. (Yes, I know that sounds like a cheesy motivational poster you'd find in a dentist's office, but stick with me here.)

There was the time I decided I needed a new challenge. Because apparently having a 12-piece metal cage in my neck, competing at the highest level, and running businesses wasn't quite enough excitement. I thought, "You know what would be fun? Learning to grapple with people twice my size!"

That's right—I decided to take up Jiu-jitsu. But I didn't just jump in randomly (okay, maybe a little randomly).

I had a plan:

1. Find a great instructor

2. Recruit a friend as my grappling partner (preferably someone bigger and stronger, because why make things easy?)

3. Commit to training twice a week

4. Accept that I was going to look like a fish flopping on land for a while

Today, I'm closing in on my blue belt—a milestone that started with "this might be a terrible idea" and transformed into "wow, I actually did that." Fun fact: only 10% of people who start Brazilian Jiu-jitsu ever earn their blue belt. I'm about to join that determined minority.

Step 1: Set Your Destination

Before you can figure out how to get somewhere, you need to know where you're going. Your goal should be specific, measurable, and maybe a little bit scary. For example:

Instead of: "I want to get fit"

Try: "I want to do a pull-up without crying" (specific and emotionally accurate)

Instead of: "I want to learn something new"

Try: "I want to learn how to not get crushed by someone twice my size in Jiu-jitsu" (specific and mildly concerning)

Step 2: Map Out the Route

Once you've set your goal, break it into smaller steps. Think of it like a road trip—you're not going to drive 1,000 miles without stopping for snacks and bathroom breaks (and probably coffee, because let's be real here).

My Jiu-jitsu roadmap looked something like this:

- Learn basic moves without accidentally choking myself

- Be methodical and go slow, this is not an explosive fitness routine.

- Master the art of tapping out gracefully

- Eventually learn enough to make my training partner question their life choices

Step 3: Stay Flexible

Life happens. Plans change. Sometimes you show up to train and your body says "Not today, Satan." That's okay. The key is to adjust your route without losing sight of your destination.

Miss a workout? Cool—do one tomorrow.

Had an entire pizza? Nice—extra fuel for training.

Got submitted 47 times in one session? Awesome—that's 47 learning opportunities!

"WHEN OBSTACLES ARISE, YOU CHANGE YOUR DIRECTION TO REACH YOUR GOAL; YOU DO NOT CHANGE YOUR DECISION TO GET THERE." - *Zig Ziglar*

The Reality Check

Here's the truth about roadmaps: sometimes you're going to take a wrong turn and end up somewhere completely unexpected. Like that time I thought I was ready for an advanced move and ended up looking like a pretzel having an existential crisis.

But here's the thing—those detours often lead to the best stories and biggest breakthroughs.

Your Action Plan

This week, try this:

1. Pick one goal that excites you (and maybe scares you a little)

2. Break it down into tiny, manageable steps

3. Tell someone about it (accountability is key)

4. Start with step one (no matter how small)

5. Celebrate every tiny victory (yes, a session without getting choked out counts as a victory)

The Plot Twist

Sometimes the best part of having a roadmap is discovering all the unexpected adventures along the way. When I started Jiu-jitsu, I thought I was just learning a new sport. Turns out I was also learning:

- Humility (nothing humbles you quite like getting trapped in someone's guard)

- Patience (with yourself and others)

- The importance of showing up (even when you're pretty sure you're going to spend most of the class tapping out)

- That the human body can bend in ways you never imagined (not always intentionally)

Your Turn: Chart Your Course

Take 15 minutes today to map out your next big goal. Remember:

- Make it specific

- Make it measurable

- Make it slightly terrifying

- Give yourself permission to modify as needed

- Keep your sense of humor handy

Because at the end of the day, success isn't just about reaching the destination—it's about all the times you got back up, laughed it off, and kept going.

And hey, if your roadmap leads you to trying something completely new? Go for it. Just maybe check the insurance coverage first. (Kidding! Kind of.)

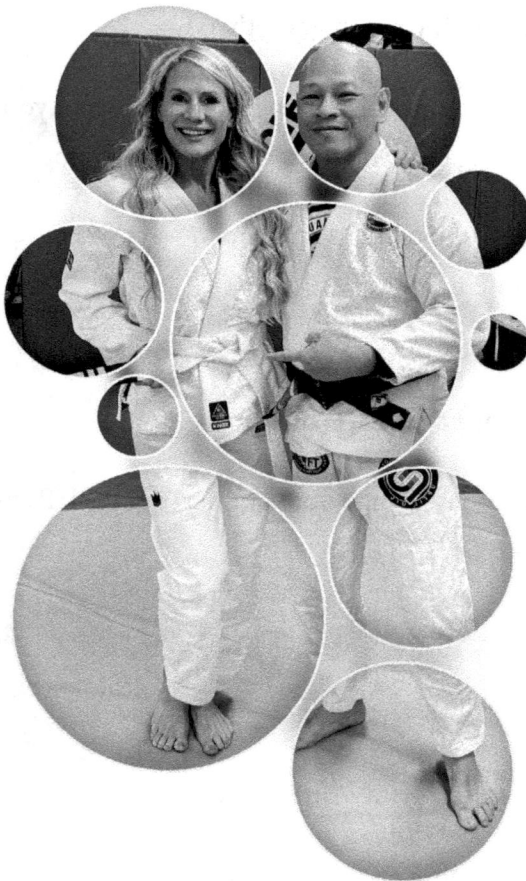

Quan Phu - Gracie Humaita Jiu-jitsu
2nd degree black belt

Your Turn:

Your Next Big Goal:

What's your next big destination, and what are the first three steps on your roadmap to get there?

_____

_____

_____

_____

_____

_____

_____

_____

_____

_____

_____

_____

What potential detours might pop up on your journey, and how will you navigate around them?

_____

_____

_____

_____

_____

_____

_____

_____

_____

_____

_____

_____

_____

_____

_____

_____

_____

_____

_____

_____

_____

_____

_____

KAYLA'S JOURNEY TO STRENGTH

One of my most meaningful impact stories involves working with Kayla, a young girl battling a severe eating disorder. When she came to me, she had already been through inpatient treatment and was at risk of relapse. Her mother reached out because she saw how I embodied both strength and joy—qualities her daughter desperately needed to reconnect with.

Rather than focusing on food, weight, or body image, we shifted the narrative to becoming "a powerful force of nature." Every session became an exploration of strength and capability. The goal wasn't to be pretty or delicate—it was to be powerful enough that "if life is going to attack you, can you defend yourself?"

This approach resonated deeply with Kayla, giving her a new lens through which to view herself. Instead of striving to be a fragile, "perfect" girl fixated on magazine ideals, she began embracing the identity of a strong, powerful female. This mindset shift was transformative—people began to notice and say things like, "Whoa, I don't want to mess with you!"

When we first started working together, what Kayla truly lacked was confidence. Over time, she began to embrace and own who she was. She stopped worrying so much about what others thought of her and stepped into the identity she had longed for—a woman who was strong, proud, driven, and viewed as "beautiful" by her *own* standards.

We worked together for about a year before she went off to a new school. The physical transformation was remarkable, but the mental transformation was profound. Kayla went from being trapped in a cycle of control and perfectionism to a young woman who understood that true strength comes from nourishing and challenging her body, not punishing it.

PART 4

The Heart of Winning Broken

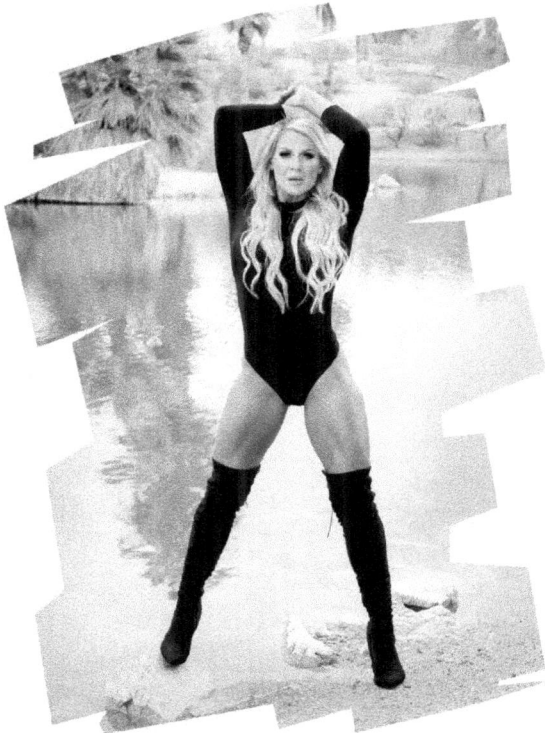

CHAPTER 11

What's Your Why?

"THE BIGGER THE CHALLENGE, THE BIGGER
THE OPPORTUNITY TO GROW"

What drives you? No, seriously—what's the thing that gets you out of bed on the days when you'd rather bury yourself under the covers? If your answer is "nothing," then we've got some work to do. And if your answer is "coffee," well, I get it. (I'm not judging—coffee's a very valid why.)

But here's the truth: having a strong "why" isn't optional. It's essential. Your why is what keeps you moving forward when progress feels slow, when life throws curveballs, and when your body is literally falling apart on stage at the 2023 Olympia.

My Why: The Boys and the Bigger Purpose

Here's the thing about that 2023 Olympia performance—it wasn't about adding another trophy to my collection (in fact: I didn't snag the win that year). It was about teaching my boys something you can't learn from a textbook. Every grimace of pain, every step on that stage with my shoulder barely cooperating—it was me showing them, when you start something, you finish it. Even when every cell in your body is begging you to walk away. Even when the "smart" choice would be to quit.

These moments remind me of what truly matters. When things get tough—whether it's a business challenge that seems impossible, a workout that's kicking my butt, or just one of those days where being a single mom feels like juggling chainsaws—I think about my boys watching me push through that pain. Because it's not just about me anymore—it's about showing them what resilience looks like in real time. And let me tell you, that's worth more than any trophy I could ever win.

Why Your Why Matters

Your why is like your GPS. Without it, you're just wandering aimlessly, hoping you end up somewhere nice. But with a clear why, you know exactly where you're headed—and you're way less likely to get stuck in a ditch.

Here's what your why does:

- **Keeps You Focused**: When distractions pop up (and they always do), your why reminds you what really matters.

- **Motivates You on Hard Days**: Let's be real—there will be days when you don't feel like showing up. Your why gives you the push you need to keep going, even when your body parts aren't exactly cooperating.

- **Makes the Struggle Worth It**: Challenges are inevitable, but when you know your why, they don't feel pointless. They feel like stepping stones.

Digging Deep: Finding Your Why

Most people stop at the surface level when they think about their why. They say things like, "I want to be healthier" or "I want to be successful." Those are great starting points, but they're not enough to sustain you when your shoulder is hanging out of its socket near the end of your routine.

Exercise: The Why Ladder

Here's how you can find your true why in three steps:

1. Write Down Your Goal: Start with something simple, like, "I want to get fit."

2. Ask Why It Matters: "Why do I want to get fit?" Your answer might be, "Because I want more energy."

3. Keep Asking Why: Take your answer and dig deeper. "Why do I want more energy?"

Maybe it's so you can keep up with your kids or feel more confident in your body or so you can do more pull-ups so that you can look like a superhero with your shirt off at the beach.

By the time you've asked why five times, you'll uncover the deeper reason that drives you. That's your why.

Using Your Why to Keep Going

Once you've found your why, the next step is using it. Write it down. Post it everywhere—your fridge, your bathroom mirror, even your car dashboard. When you feel like giving up, let your why remind you why you started.

And remember, your why doesn't have to involve anything as dramatic as finishing a world-class competition with multiple injuries. It just has to matter deeply to you. Because when it really matters, you'll find strength you didn't know you had.

Bonus: Whitney's "Why" Ritual

I want to positively impact people. Each morning, I send messages to people I'm thinking about. Sometimes it's a meaningful note, sometimes it's just an off-humor meme—it's the connection that matters.

Every day, I also visualize my why. I think about my boys, their smiles, and the kind of life I want to build for them. Then I say out loud, "This is why I do what I do." It might sound cheesy, but it works. Try it—I dare you.

Your Turn: Reflect on Your Why

Take 15 minutes today to journal about your why. Start with your goal, then ask yourself why it matters—again and again—until you get to the heart of it. And remember: your why doesn't have to be perfect. It just has to matter to you.

Celebrating Your Why

Here's the fun part: once you've found your why, celebrate it. Maybe it's a toast with friends, a happy dance in your living room, or a Dr. Pepper® shake from Whataburger®. Whatever it is, make it a moment. Because your why is worth celebrating.

Even if you're celebrating with an ice pack on your shoulder.

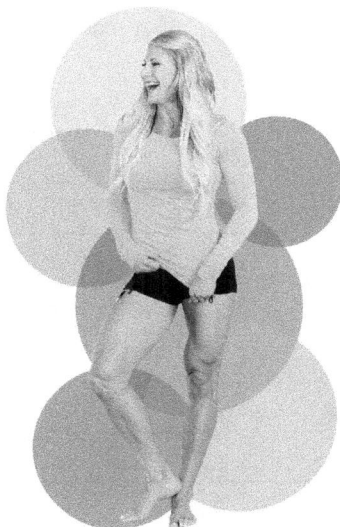

Your Turn:

What is your goal?

_____

_____

_____

_____

_____

Why?

_____

_____

_____

_____

Why?

_____

_____

_____

_____

Why?

_____

_____

_____

_____

Why

_____

_____

_____

_____

Why?

_____

_____

_____

_____

My WHY is:

_____

_____

_____

_____

_____

_____

_____

CHAPTER 12

Identity Is Everything

"THE BEST PROJECT YOU COULD EVER WORK ON IS YOU." – *Karon Waddell*

Here's a question for you: who do you think you are? And no, I don't mean that in the sassy reality TV way where someone's about to throw a drink in someone else's face. I mean, when was the last time you dreamed as big as you did when you were a kid?

Remember those days, when someone asked what you wanted to be when you grew up, and you'd say "A superhero-astronaut-veterinarian who also runs a cookie factory on the moon"? And nobody told you that was impossible because, well, why crush a perfectly good dream?

The Power of Unlimited Thinking

Let me take you back to a moment in my life when everything fell apart. Post-divorce, standing in the middle of what felt like ground zero of my old life, I had a choice to make. I could either stay in the rubble, or I could do something crazy—like reimagine my entire life.

That's when it hit me: when was the last time I felt truly unlimited? When did I start listening to all the "you can'ts" and "you shouldn'ts"? So I did something radical. I channeled my inner eight-year-old, the one who thought anything was possible, and I asked myself: "If no one could tell me no, what would I do?"

Turns out, that inner eight-year-old had some pretty wild ideas. And you know what? Some of them weren't half bad.

> "BE YOURSELF AND YOU CAN BE ANYTHING."
> – *Einstein*

Your Identity Shapes Your Actions

Think about it: if you believe you're "not a morning person," are you going to wake up early for a workout? About as likely as my dog learning to do taxes. If you believe you're "not disciplined," are you going to stick to your goals? Probably not.

But what if you started seeing yourself differently? What if instead of:

- "I'm not a morning person" → "I'm learning to embrace the sunrise"

- "I'm not athletic" → "I'm on a journey to move my body in new ways"

- "I can't do that" → "I can't do that YET"

See what I did there? Same person, different story.

Rewriting Your Story

The good news? Your identity isn't set in stone. You can rewrite it anytime you want. It's like being the author of your own superhero origin story, minus the radioactive spider bites (though I'm not ruling those out entirely).

Step 1: Get Honest

Take a good, hard look at the story you're telling yourself. Are you saying things like:

- "I'm not good at this"

- "I could never do that"

- "That's not who I am"

Write those thoughts down—not because they're true, but because we're about to flip them on their head like a gymnast who's had way too much sugar.

Step 2: Flip the Script

For every negative statement, write a new one that reflects who you want to become:

- Instead of "I'm not disciplined" → "I'm building discipline every day"

- Instead of "I'm not fit" → "I'm getting stronger with every workout"

- Instead of "I'm too old for this" → "I'm just getting started"

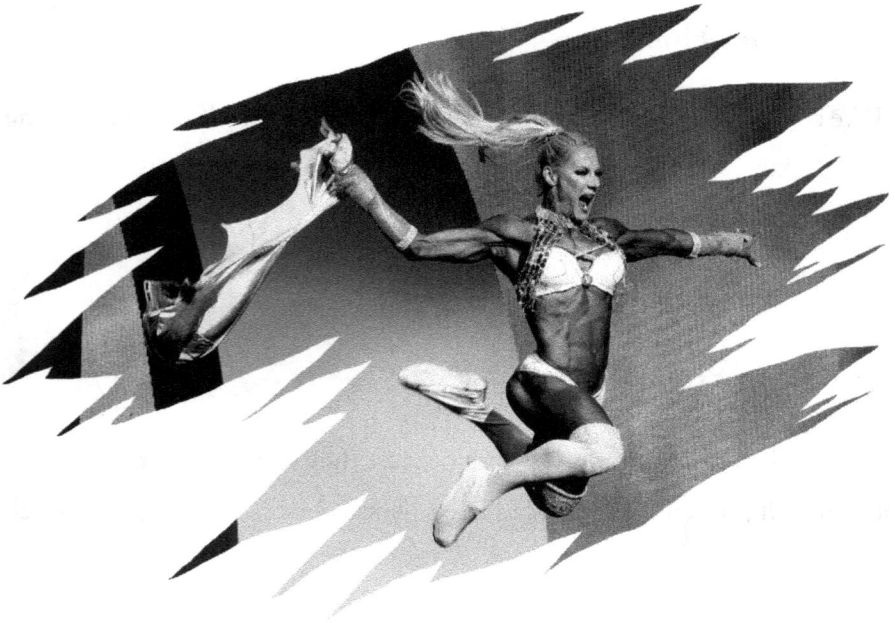

Step 3: Start Small

You don't have to overhaul your life overnight. That's like trying to eat an entire cake in one bite—messy, probably ill-advised, and likely to give you a stomach ache. Instead, pick one small action that aligns with your new identity.

The "I Am" Effect

There's something powerful about starting a sentence with "I am." It's like casting a spell, but instead of turning someone into a frog, you're transforming yourself into who you want to be.

My favorite "I am" statements:

- "I am a work in progress, and that's okay"

- "I am resilient, even when life gets messy"

- "I am someone who shows up for myself every single day"

- "I am the kind of person who tries new things, even if I look ridiculous doing them"

Real-Life Example: The Client Who Found Her "I Am"

Meet Lisa (let's call her that because, well, that's her name). She came to me feeling completely defeated. Her words? "I've always been the chubby girl, and that's just who I am."

We started small. Her first "I am" statement was simply "I am trying." (Hey, it's a start!) But over time, those statements got bolder:

- "I am strong"

- "I am confident"

- "I am a total badass"

Six months later, Lisa wasn't just hitting her fitness goals—she was strutting around the gym like she owned the place. That's the power of rewriting your story.

Your Turn: Own Your Identity

1. Write down three "I am" statements that align with who you want to become

2. Ask yourself: What would this person do today?

3. Take one small action that matches your new identity

4. Repeat until it feels natural (or at least less awkward)

Remember: No one else gets to decide who you are. Not your past, not your circumstances, not even that one person who said you'd never make it (looking at you, Karen from high school).

You get to decide. So decide to be unstoppable. Decide to dream big. Decide to be the person your eight-year-old self would think is totally awesome.

Because at the end of the day, the only permission you need to be amazing is your own.

Now, if you'll excuse me, I need to go work on that cookie factory on the moon idea. Hey, you never know...

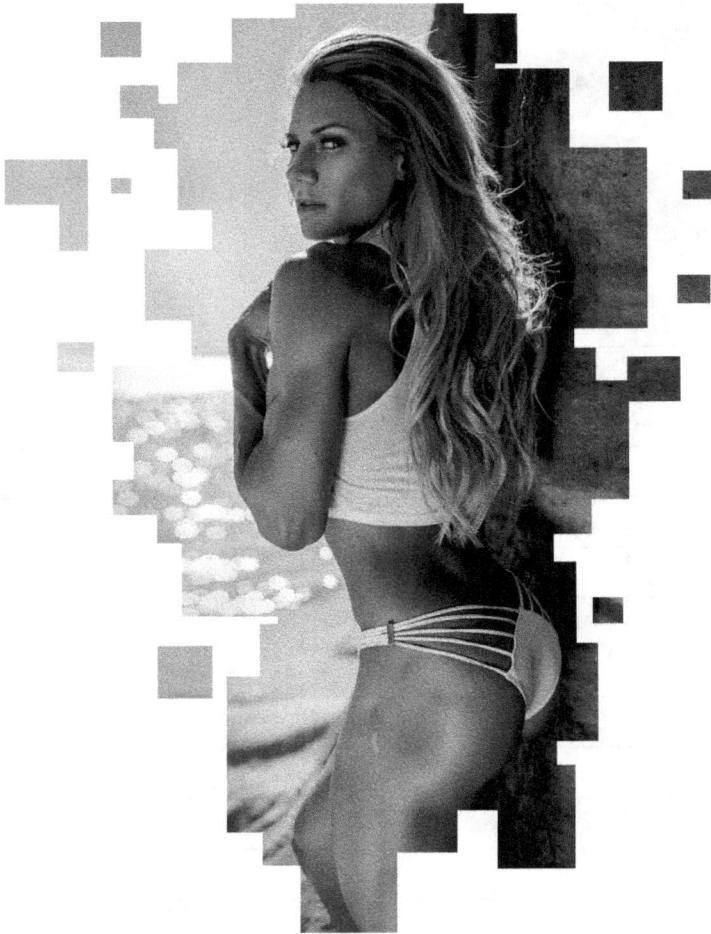

Your Turn:

Re-write your I Am Statements:

_____
_____
_____
_____
_____
_____
_____
_____
_____
_____
_____
_____
_____
_____
_____

Who do you want to become?

_____

_____

_____

_____

_____

_____

_____

_____

_____

_____

_____

_____

_____

_____

_____

_____

_____

_____

_____

_____

_____

_____

_____

_____

CHAPTER 13

Celebrate the Journey

"AFTER A WHILE I LOOKED IN THE MIRROR AND REALIZED, WOW AFTER ALL THOSE HURTS, SCARS, AND BRUISES, AFTER ALL OF THOSE TRIALS, I REALLY MADE IT THROUGH. I DID IT. I SURVIVED THAT WHICH WAS SUPPOSED TO KILL ME. SO I STRAIGHTENED MY CROWN..AND WALKED AWAY LIKE A BOSS." – *Unknown*

Here's a mistake I see people make all the time: they wait. They wait until they hit the big milestone, achieve the perfect result, or cross some imaginary finish line before they let themselves celebrate. And you know what happens? They miss out on all the joy along the way—including the character-building moments like breaking your nose three times and having to reset it yourself. (Yes, really. And yes, we're going to talk about it.)

The last time I broke my nose, I face-planted during a routine practice (because apparently, my face needed a closer inspection of the floor). I popped up and immediately thought, "Oh great, broke it again." But here's the fun part—instead of panicking, I went into DIY plastic surgeon mode.

Now, most people would rush to a doctor. Me? I grabbed a metal rod and, while still in shock (thank goodness for that adrenaline window), decided to play amateur rhinoplasty. Why? Because the previous breaks left it crooked, and I figured, "Hey, free alignment opportunity!" Is this advisable? Probably not. Did it work? Actually, yes. Do I recommend it? Absolutely not—but it makes for a great story.

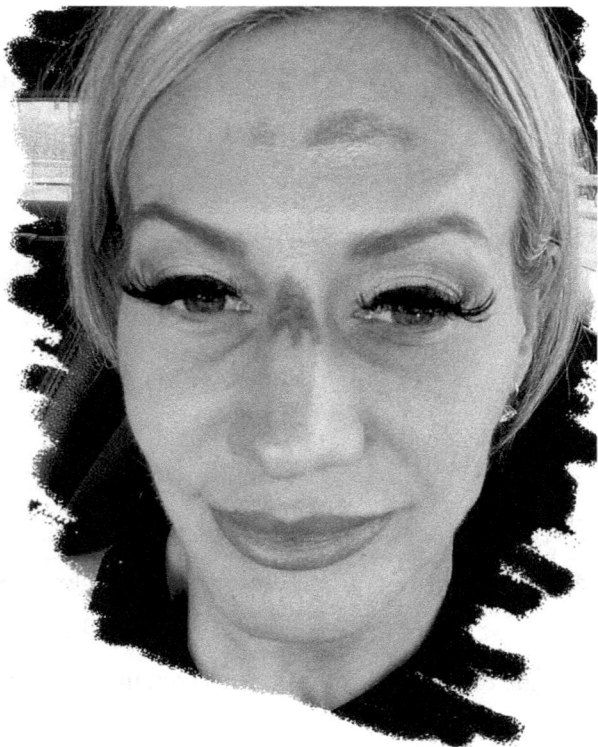

The Art of Celebrating Everything

Life isn't about waiting for the perfect moment—it's about finding the perfect moment in the imperfect situation. Like when my broken nose led to my best MacGyver impression, or when battle scars became badges of honor.

Take my wrists, for instance. They don't look like normal wrists anymore because I've broken them so many times. For years, I tried to hide them, feeling self-conscious about how they looked. But you know what? These aren't flaws—they're evidence that I showed up, that I tried, that I lived.

Why Celebrating Matters

Here's the thing about celebration: it's not just about having fun (though that's a pretty great bonus). It's about:

1. **Acknowledging Progress**: Every step forward counts, even if that step is just learning how to reset your own nose. (Again, please don't try this at home.)

2. **Building Momentum**: When you celebrate small wins, you're more likely to keep going. It's like leaving yourself a trail of party breadcrumbs.

3. **Changing Your Perspective**: Instead of seeing scars as imperfections, you start seeing them as your superhero origin story.

The Small Stuff Is Actually the Big Stuff

I say, have fun and accessorize your injuries! For example, when I injured my AC joint and collarbone, I wore a fancy little Dutch hat on it. (I wish I had a photo of that!) Instead of trying to hide it, I even drew a smiley face on it. People would stare, and I'd say, "Yeah, it looks ugly, but he's smiling at you!" It turned an awkward moment into a conversation starter.

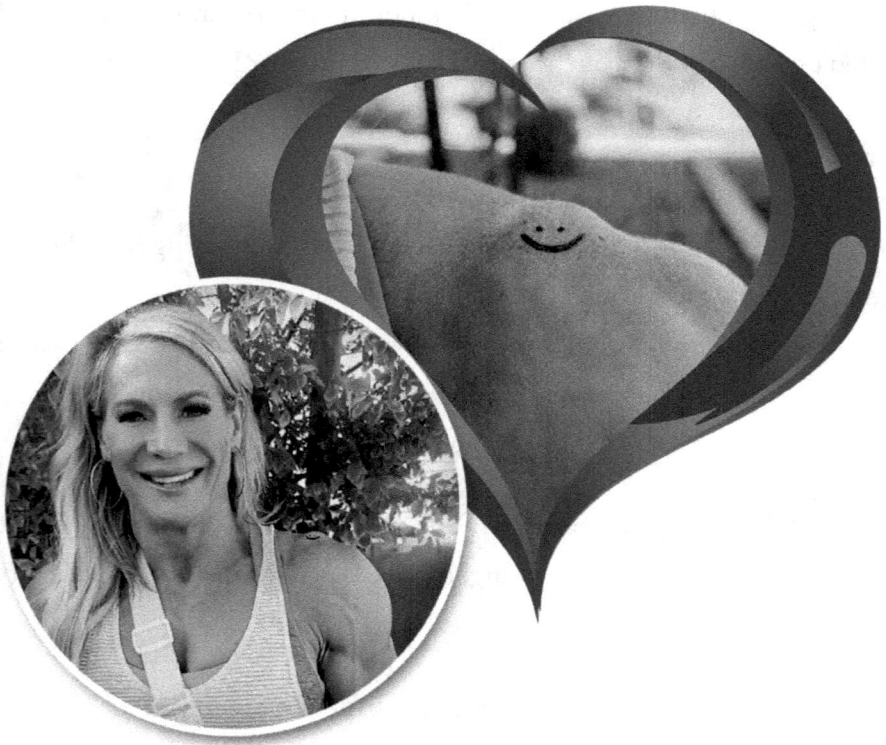

That's what celebration is about—finding the smile in the struggle, the victory in the visible scars.

Ways to Celebrate That Don't Require Medical Attention

1. **The Daily Victory Dance**: Did something good happen? Dance! Did something bad happen? Dance anyway! (Just watch out for low ceilings.)

2. **The Gratitude Flip**: Take something that seems negative and find its silver lining. Like how my crooked nose finally got straightened out... by another break. Talk about unexpected blessings!

3. **The Progress Photo**: Document your journey—scars, bruises, victories, and all. They're not imperfections; they're your story's illustrations.

Real-Life Celebration Stories

Remember when I dislocated my shoulder during that Olympia performance? After it was all over, you know what I did? My friends took me out to celebrate with a "My Shoulder's Back Where It Belongs" sort of party. Because if you can't laugh at life's plot twists, what's the point?

Celebrating Through the Setbacks

Here's a secret: sometimes the best celebrations happen on the hardest days. Like when I had to perform with a broken leg and turned my "don't let them see you limping" walk into a signature strut. Work with what you've got, right?

Your Turn: Create Your Celebration Ritual

Think about something you're currently struggling with. Now, find one thing about it worth celebrating. Maybe it's:

- Your resilience in facing it

- The lesson you're learning

- The fact that you're still standing (or limping fabulously)

- The story you'll get to tell later

The Trophy Case of Life

You know those perfect trophy cases with shiny medals all lined up? Life's not like that. It's messier, more interesting, and way more fun. Your trophy case might include:

- A crooked nose with character

- Wrists that tell stories

- Battle scars that make you uniquely you

- And maybe a few actual trophies (dents and all)

Celebrate every victory, honor every scar—transform your struggles into triumphs at **EmpoweringLegends.com**.

Share your wins on Social Media using **#WinBroken** so we can we celebrate victories together!

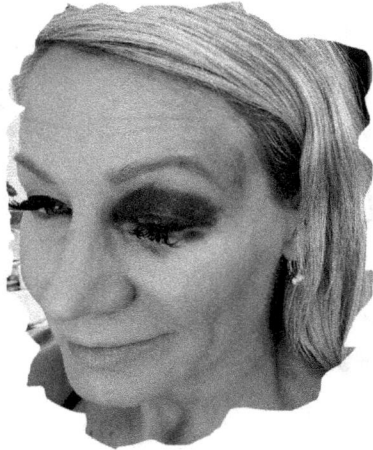

Oops, I did it again...

The Final Word on Celebration

Remember: You don't have to wait until everything's perfect to celebrate. Celebrate the mess. Celebrate the struggle. Celebrate the fact that you're still going, still trying, still showing up—even if showing up sometimes means drawing smiley faces on protruding bones or adding tons of bling to your neck brace.

Because at the end of the day, it's not about how many times you broke your nose—it's about how many times you got back up, fixed it (preferably with professional medical help), and kept going.

Now go celebrate something. Anything. Everything. Just maybe keep the DIY medical procedures to a minimum.

"YOUR FUTURE IS CREATED BY WHAT YOU DO TODAY, NOT TOMORROW." - *Robert Kiyosaki*

Your Turn:

What 'imperfect' victory deserves celebration?

_____

_____

_____

_____

_____

_____

_____

_____

_____

_____

_____

_____

_____

_____

How did a setback-turned-success make you stronger?

Ashley: Breaking Barriers in Mexico

A shley's story demonstrates how determination can overcome seemingly impossible obstacles. Training to be a professional figure competitor is challenging enough with ideal conditions - Ashley had to do it in Mexico with minimal equipment and numerous cultural barriers.

She was training in gyms that didn't have basic equipment, and when they did, she often faced resistance. Once, she was actually thrown out of a gym for running on the treadmill - they said members weren't allowed to run because it would "break the equipment." Getting competition-ready requires precise nutrition, but she couldn't just go to the store for staples like lean protein - everything had to be specially sourced and delivered.

We had to get creative with her training. When traditional gym equipment wasn't available, we utilized beach stairs for cardio and we developed innovative bodyweight routines. What impressed me most was her adaptability - when one approach didn't work, she never used it as an excuse. Instead, she'd say, "Okay, what can we try next?"

The physical transformation was remarkable given the circumstances. We had to be extremely precise about shaping her physique with limited tools. When regular exercises weren't possible, we'd analyze videos of her movement patterns and create alternative exercises to target specific muscle groups.

But more than just changing her body, Ashley proved that with enough determination, you can find a way to reach your goals regardless of your circumstances. Her journey taught me that there's always a way if you're willing to be creative and persistent enough to find it.

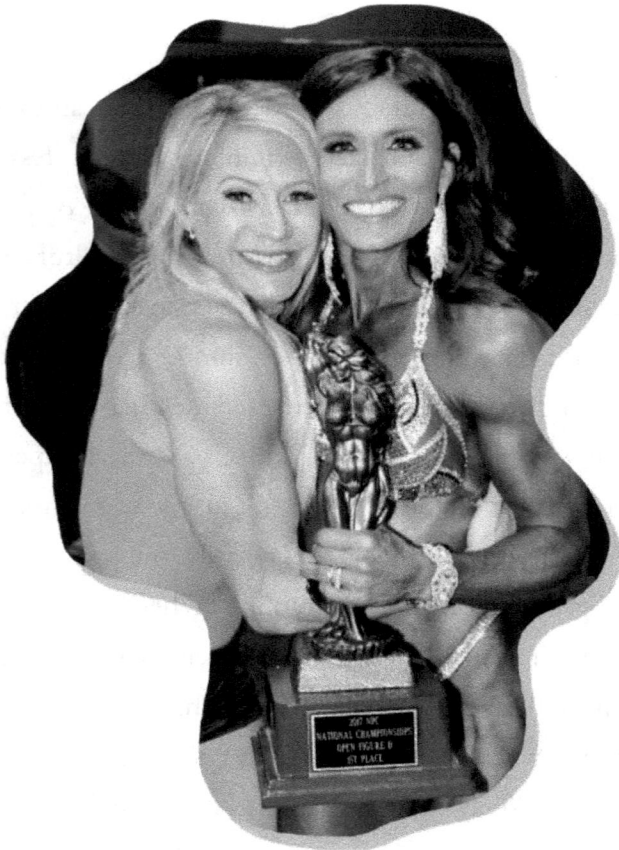

PART 5

Bonus Content and Reflections

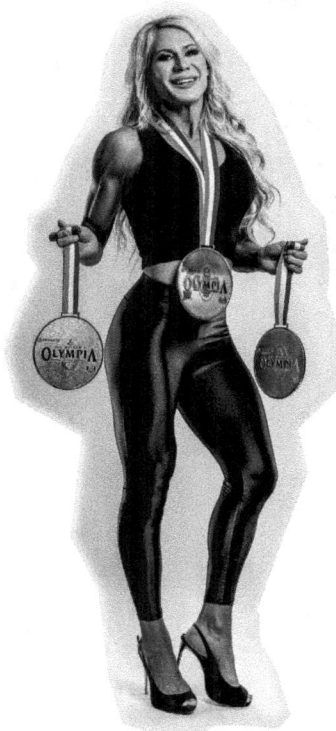

CHAPTER 14

A Day in the Life of Whitney Jones

"FOCUS ON PROBLEMS, YOU'LL HAVE MORE PROBLEMS. WHEN YOU FOCUS ON POSSIBILITIES, YOU'LL HAVE MORE OPPORTUNITIES. DREAM. WISH. MAKE IT HAPPEN." – *Whitney Jones*

Horoscope Time (Yes, Really)

Here's my guilty pleasure confession: I read my horoscope every morning. Not just one—I have multiple horoscope apps. If one says something I don't like, I just keep reading others until I find one that matches my plans for the day. Is this scientifically sound? Absolutely not. Do I do it anyway? You bet your cosmic energy I do.

The Morning Messages

Each morning, I think through my list of people who need some love and support—who's going through something tough, who needs a pick-me-up. It's my way of starting the day by thinking of others. Because nothing says "I care" like bombarding someone with inspirational memes and emojis at 6 AM.

Work, Coaching, and Controlled Chaos

This is the heart of my day. Between running my businesses, coaching clients, and managing all the behind-the-scenes details, my schedule looks like someone threw a calendar at a fan. But here's the thing: I wouldn't trade it for anything.

Pro tip: When you're juggling a million things, humor is your best friend. Like that time I accidentally joined a Zoom meeting with my camera on (while nobody else had theirs on) in pajamas, no makeup, and hair that looked like I'd been electrocuted—all while walking on a treadmill. Did I panic? Nope. I just announced that I was taking the "work-out from home" concept to a whole new level.

Gym Time (Where the Magic/Mayhem Happens)

By now, I'm ready to hit the gym. My workouts are my happy place—a time to focus, sweat, and remind myself that I'm stronger than my excuses (and occasionally my common sense).

Some days it's heavy lifting, other days it's HIIT (High Intensity Interval Training) , and sometimes it's me trying to convince my training partners to join me in some wild experiment that probably belongs on "World's Craziest Workout Fails." Safety first, viral video potential second.

The Mom Hustle

After the gym, it's time to switch hats and become 'Mom Whitney.' This used to involve wrangling two boys and playing personal chauffeur to get them everywhere on time. These days, they drive themselves, which is both a blessing and terrifying. (Is it too late to go back to the days when my biggest worry was them eating Play-Doh?) Now my time is filled with cheering at their sporting events, tackling homework together, making dinner, and—my favorite part—laughing with my boys.

Daily Mental Cross-Training

Remember my dad having dementia? That's why I do mental crossword puzzles every night. Think of it as cross-training for my brain. Though sometimes I wonder if doing CrossFit-style workouts while attempting crossword puzzles would be more efficient. (Note to self: Put that on the list to try.)

Evening Wind-Down

Before bed, I always:

- Do something for my mental health (like crossword puzzles)

- Scroll through social media for laughs

- Send memes to friends

- Plan tomorrow's chaos

- Set alarms that "Tomorrow Whitney" will definitely not appreciate

The Reality Check

Here's the truth about my day: it never goes according to plan. Ever. But that's okay because:

1. Plans are just suggestions

2. Chaos is more interesting anyway

3. The best stories come from the days that go completely off the rails

Whitney's Favorite Daily Mantras

1. "You don't HAVE to, you GET to." (Even when what you "get to" do is take Tylenol® after a concussion – I've had nine!)

2. "Progress over perfection" (Unless we're talking about snacks—then perfection matters.)

3. "Let's do it" – take risks, be bold, seize the opportunity, because regret is a b*tch.

4. "Everything is figure-out-able" (Yes, even DIY medical procedures—though please don't)

Remember: Life doesn't care about your plans. The key is to roll with it, laugh through it, and maybe keep a bag of chips handy. Because at the end of the day, it's not about having the perfect schedule—it's about making the chaos look good.

And if all else fails, just pretend whatever just happened was totally intentional. Works every time. (Except maybe that time I split my pants during a high kick demonstration. That one was harder to play off.)

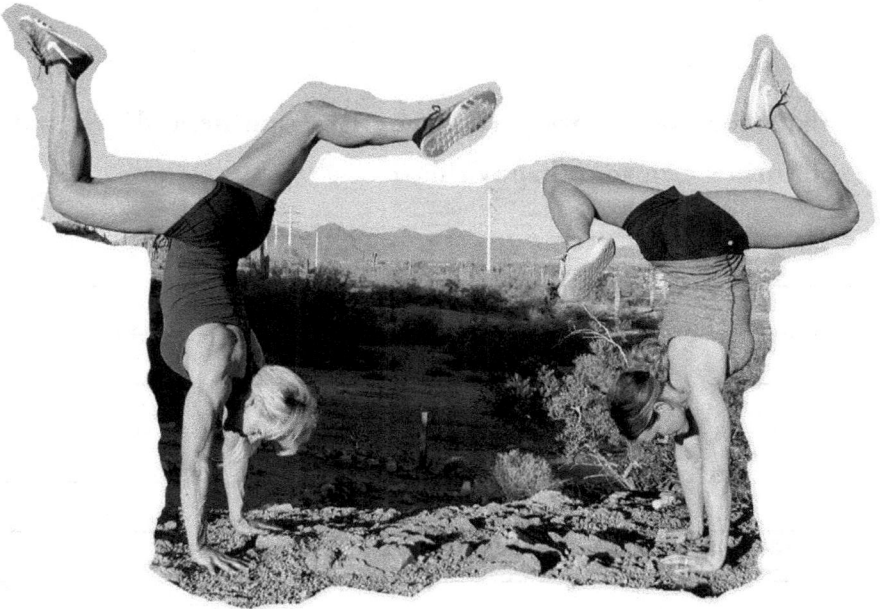

Your Turn:

What's the most chaotic part of your daily routine, and how could you turn it into your 'happy time'?

_____

_____

_____

_____

_____

_____

_____

_____

_____

_____

_____

_____

_____

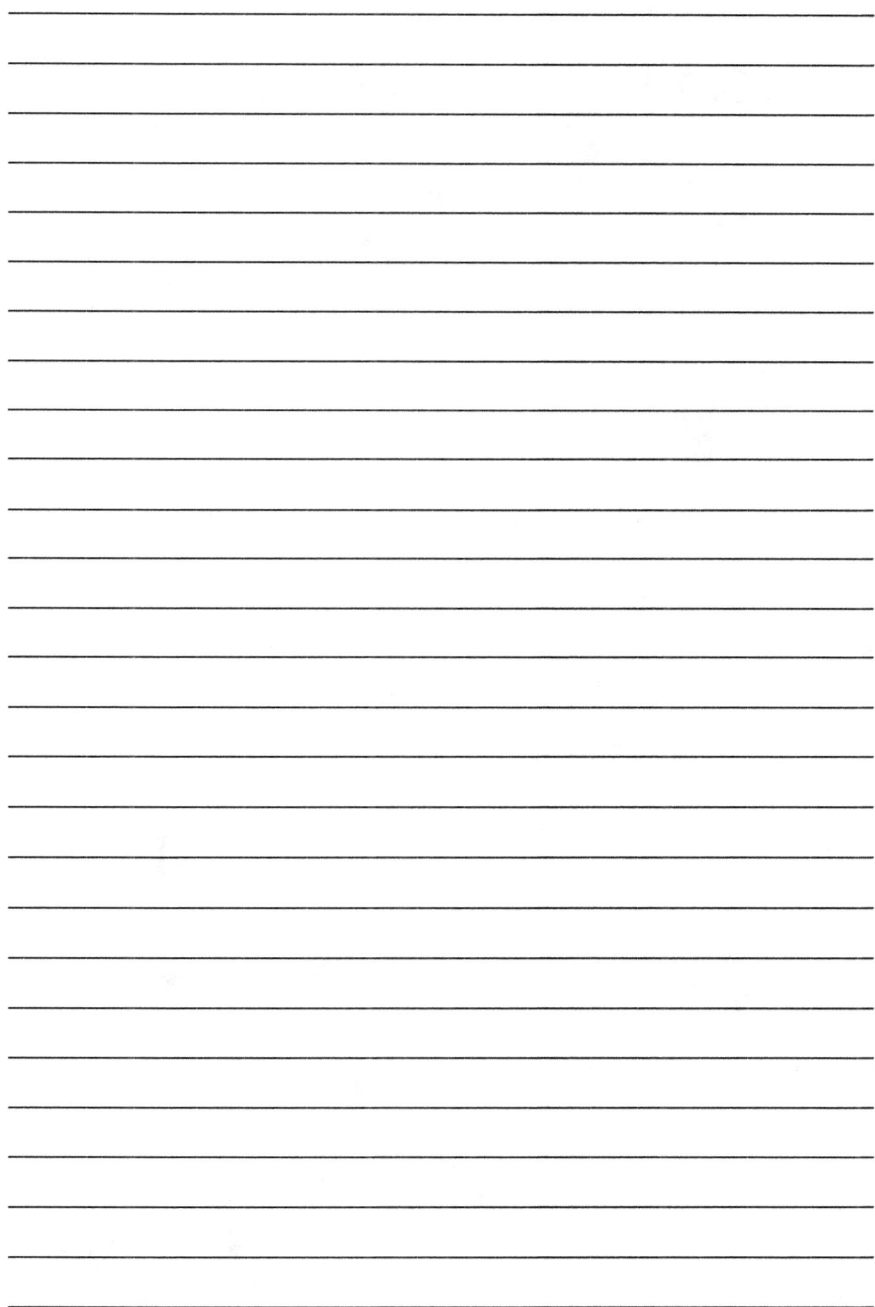

WHY YOU SHOULD ALWAYS HAVE A SPOTTER

Surprise! You Found the Secret Chapter

Okay, so if you're wondering why this chapter isn't in the table of contents, here's the deal: it's because I'm Whitney Jones, and if you haven't figured it out by now, I don't exactly color inside the lines. I mean, come on—I'm the girl who reset her own nose (three times!), competed with a broken leg, and once accidentally started a social media riot with the wrong emoji. Did you really think I'd write a book that follows all the rules?

Ok, so now I have to share the embarrassing emoji story. There I was, driving back from Tucson, wanting to celebrate this incredibly sweet girl who I had just performed with at a charity event. In my heart, I thought I was commenting on her Instagram post with a "You're #1!" message, accompanied by what I thought was the pointing-up emoji.

Instead—thanks to my less-than-perfect vision and speeding thumbs—I ended up posting **four middle finger emojis.** (In my defense, the middle finger emoji does look a lot like the pointing-up one.)

It wasn't until my friend texted "Uh, Whitney... did you mean to do that?" that I realized my supportive celebration looked more like an angry protest. Cue me frantically pulling over on the highway to edit a post that made it look like I was hating on this amazing young girl. Not exactly the "way to go, kiddo!" message I was aiming for. Maybe don't post emojis while driving, and definitely double-check which finger you're pointing to the sky.

Think of this chapter as the equivalent of finding a $20 bill in your coat pocket that you forgot about. You weren't expecting it, but you're definitely not mad about it.

And yes, I know what you're thinking: "Whitney, you can't just add random chapters that aren't in the table of contents!" Watch me. Because this is my book, and if I can figure out how to perform a routine with a dislocated shoulder, I can definitely sneak in a bonus chapter.

Consider this your reward for actually reading the book instead of just looking at the pictures. Now, buckle up, because if I'm breaking the rules of book structure, you know this chapter's going to be good...

Christmas Adventure Ride

Here's something you should know about me: I keep my Christmas tree up all year. Yes, you read that right. In July, when most people are thinking about beach towels and barbecues, I've got a 16-foot reminder of holiday cheer twinkling away in my living room. Think of it as my personal protest against seasonal limitations. Why should joy be confined to December?

Every November, I re-theme it—because one theme per year just isn't enough when you're committed to year-round festivity. Usually, my boys help with this process. They're both over six feet tall and built like linebackers, which comes in handy when you're decorating something that could double as a small redwood.

But this particular day, they weren't around. And I, in my infinite wisdom, decided that this was absolutely the perfect time to redecorate the top of the tree. Solo. Because apparently, having a metal cage in my neck and a history of breaking every bone in my body wasn't enough of a warning sign.

So there I am, perched at the top of a ladder that's definitely meant for someone with a little more common sense, trying to arrange an elaborate topper that would make Martha Stewart jealous. The ladder starts wobbling—you know, that moment when your life flashes before your eyes and you think, "Well, this is going to make a great story... if I survive."

I made a split-second decision that would have made my insurance agent cry. I hugged that tree like my life depended on it (which, let's be honest, it kind of did).

What followed was less "graceful descent" and more "National Lampoon's Christmas Vacation meets Olympic luge." I slid down all sixteen feet of that tree, probably setting some kind of speed record for vertical pine tree descent. The branches whooshed past my face like I was starring in my own holiday action movie.

When I finally reached the bottom, I just sat there, having what I like to call a "life evaluation moment." Was anything broken? Nope. Was the tree still standing? Somehow, yes. Was it about to fall over and crush me? Luckily, no. Was this going to stop me from doing something equally questionable in the future? Also no.

I stood up, brushed off the artificial pine needles (as well as the glass from the lights and ornaments – I'll spare you the gory details), flipped my hair, and pretended this was all part of my master plan. Because when life gives you an impromptu tree slide, you style it out.

The tree? Still stands proud year-round. The ladder? We've come to an understanding—it judges me silently, and I pretend not to notice. And my boys? They mysteriously always seem to be available for tree decorating now. Funny how that works.

Remember folks: Sometimes the best stories start with "This seemed like a good idea at the time." Just maybe have someone spot you. Or don't. I'm not your mom. But I am the unofficial world record holder for fastest descent of a Christmas tree, so there's that.

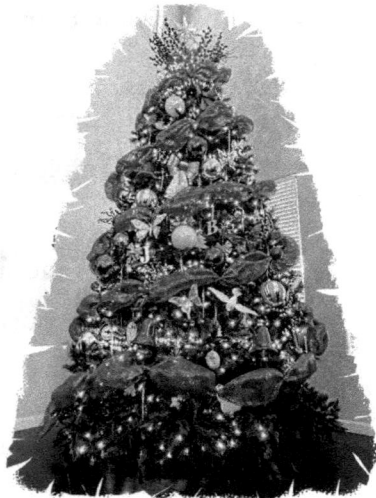

CHAPTER 15

Lessons from Falling Flat on My Face (Literally)

EVEN IF YOU FALL ON YOUR FACE, YOU'RE STILL MOVING FORWARD." - *Victor Kiam*

I f there's one thing I've mastered in life, it's the art of the face plant. And I'll tell you, I've turned it into an Olympic-level sport. Not that there's a Face Plant category at the Olympia (yet), but if there was, I'd definitely be a contender for the title.

There I was at the Toronto Pro in the middle of my routine, feeling like a superhero, when suddenly—BAM! Face meets floor in what could be called a "surprise gravity check." The crowd gasps. The judges wince. And there I am, thinking, "Well, this isn't part of the choreography."

But that's just the warm-up act. Now I will share some of my greatest hits (literally) from the "Oops Files."

The Hawaii Pro Bikini Crisis

Here's a pro tip: always triple-check your competition wear. I learned this the hard way at the Hawaii Pro when my bikini decided to malfunction right in the middle of my model turns. *Pop* goes the bikini, and there I am, trying to maintain my composure while also maintaining my modesty.

Did I panic? Maybe a little. But I channeled my inner quick-change artist, managed to step to the side when it was my turn, finished my poses (albeit a bit more carefully), and somehow pulled it off. The best part? I ended up winning that show. Because sometimes it's not about what goes wrong—it's about how creatively you handle it.

The Extension Extraction

I'm being interviewed on camera by a major fitness magazine. I'm feeling confident, looking good, but trying to move my hair out of my face—when suddenly one of my tape-in hair extension decides it wants to make a solo appearance. It just casually detaches itself and sticks to my finger while I was mid-sentence like it's making a break for freedom.

I'm trying to play it cool, as my extension is just hanging there like, "Surprise! I'm not going anywhere!" as I'm trying to shake it off. The best part? We were live. So I did what any professional would do—I held it up and announced, "And for my next trick..." Sometimes you just have to lean into the chaos. The lady conducting the interview was horrified and not sure what to do, definitely not laughing, but I was.

The Great Spelling Bee Incident of Sixth Grade

Some embarrassing moments are like fine wine—they get better (or at least funnier) with age. Take my sixth-grade spelling bee, for instance. My mom bought me new jeans from Marshalls for the big event because, you know, spelling champions need to look sharp. What we didn't count on was the zipper being about as reliable as New Year's diet resolutions.

There I was, on stage in front of the entire school, ready to spell my way to glory, when suddenly, everyone started giggling and trying to tell me something. Fast forward to the mortifying moment when they had to announce over the mic, "Whitney, your zipper's down."

I had to walk off stage, fix it, and come back. But because the universe has a sense of humor, the humiliation didn't end there—they accidentally (but cruelly) put the photo in the yearbook.

Life Lessons from Face Plants

Here's what I've learned from my various encounters with gravity, wardrobes, and social media mishaps:

1. **Recovery Is an Art Form**: Sometimes it's not about preventing the fall—it's about how fabulously you get back up.

2. **Humor Is Your Best Accessory**: When your extension is trying to escape during a live interview, you might as well make it part of the show.

3. **Always Have a Backup Plan**: Whether it's a costume, a routine, or a social media post, always have Plan B ready.

The Whitney Recovery Method

1. **Assess the Situation**: Is it a real crisis or just an embarrassing moment? Like, are we talking broken bone or broken zipper?

2. **Choose Your Response**: You can either let it defeat you or turn it into a story worth telling. (Hint: The story option is way more fun.)

3. **Add Some Flair**: If you're going to recover, do it with style. Strike a pose, crack a joke, or just smile like you meant to do that all along.

The Real Lesson Here

Life isn't about being perfect—it's about being perfectly okay with being imperfect. It's about getting up after every fall, laughing after every wardrobe malfunction, and remembering that sometimes the best stories start with "This wasn't part of the plan."

So the next time you find yourself in an awkward situation, just remember: somewhere out there, I'm probably doing something equally embarrassing, but with jazz hands.

Because at the end of the day, it's not about how many times you fall—it's about how many times you get back up, keep moving, and make everyone wonder if that face plant was actually part of the choreography.

(Spoiler alert: It never is. But hey, we can pretend.)

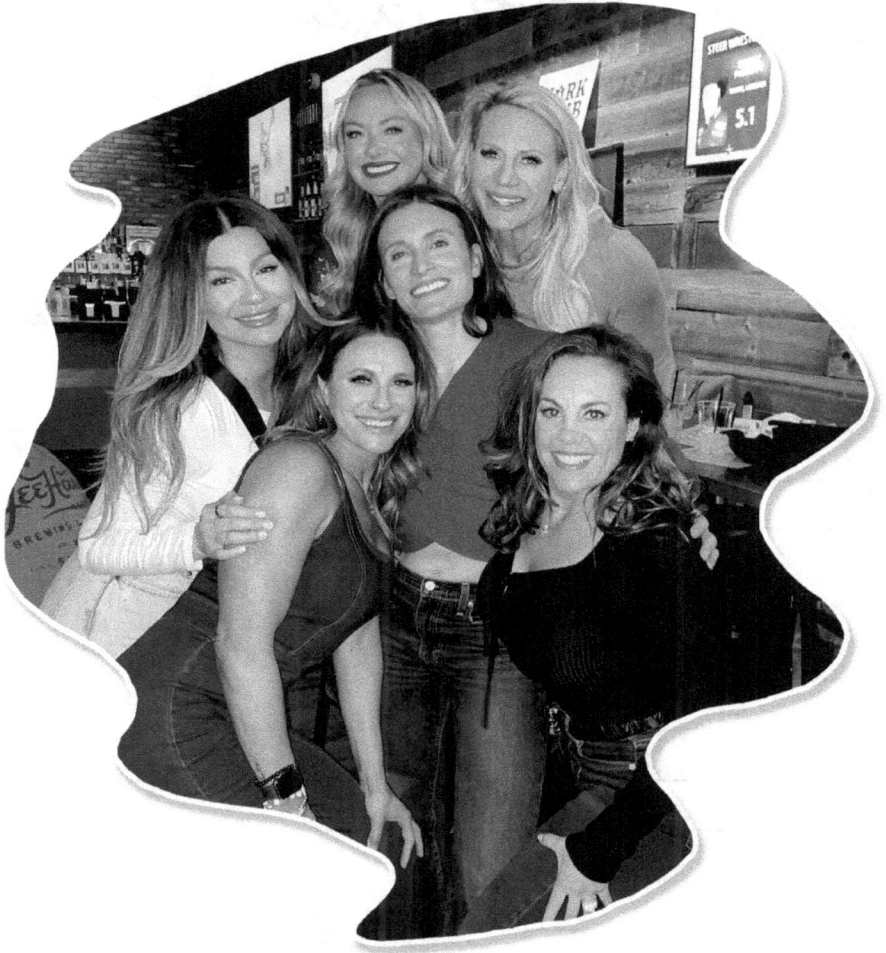

When Life Knocks You Down, Friends Pick You Up

Your Turn:

What moments can you laugh about now that you couldn't in the moment?

_____

_____

_____

_____

_____

_____

_____

_____

_____

_____

_____

_____

_____

_____

With the wisdom you have now, how would you approach that situation differently?

_____

_____

_____

_____

_____

_____

_____

_____

_____

_____

_____

_____

_____

_____

_____

_____

_____

_____

_____

_____

_____

_____

_____

CHAPTER 16

How to Build Unstoppable Confidence

"IF YOU DON'T GO AFTER WHAT YOU WANT, YOU'LL NEVER HAVE IT. IF YOU DON'T ASK, THE ANSWER IS ALWAYS NO. IF YOU DON'T STEP FORWARD YOU'RE ALWAYS IN THE SAME PLACE."

There was this one time I was facing a lion in Africa. I was on safari, rocking a "Slay All Day" t-shirt (the irony was not lost on me), when our guide started tossing steaks to keep the lions interested so we could get the classic tourist photos. My pulse was racing as we stood inches away from these ravenous beasts.

Later, we encountered some younger lions, and one actually swiped at me! The guides kept calmly repeating, "Don't move, stay calm," while I was internally screaming, "You're absolutely crazy—get me out of here!"

We had to strategize for about 10 agonizing minutes to figure out how to get me out safely. Let's just say, it was the most nerve-wracking moment of my life.

But here's the thing - they were right. Running wasn't an option. I had to face my fear head-on and trust the process. That experience taught me something crucial about confidence: it's not about being fearless—it's about being scared and doing it anyway. That lesson reinforced everything I'd learned, just like the skydiving experience. Suddenly, when someone asked, "Hey, can you try this new skill?" or "Want to attempt this never-before-seen move?" I would tell myself, "Well, I faced a lion... this can't be scarier than that, right?

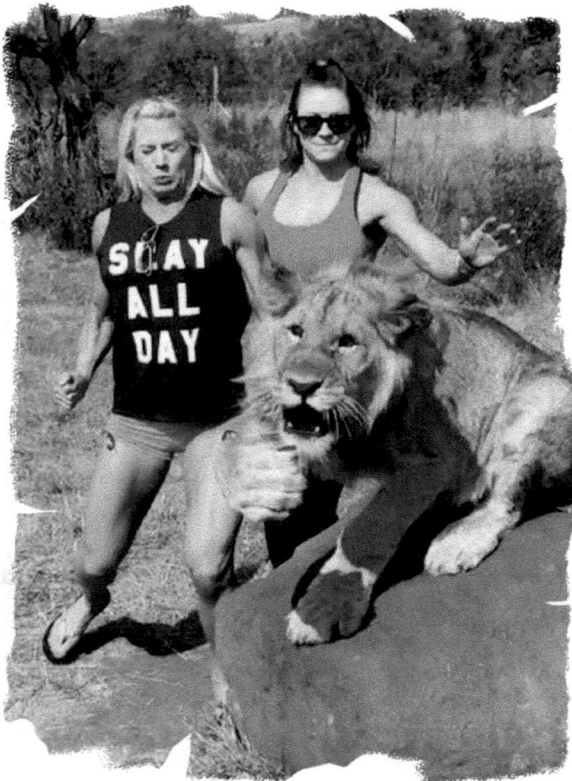

Building Confidence Through Action

Want to know the real secret to confidence? It's action. Small steps, big leaps, and sometimes a few face-plants along the way. Here's how I build mine:

1. **Start Small**:

   - Speak up in a meeting

   - Try out a new sport or activity

   - Wear that outfit you've been saving for "someday"

   - Maybe don't start with skydiving (learn from my questionable decision-making)

2. **Celebrate Everything**:

   - Did you try something new? That's a win

   - Did you fail but get back up? Also a win

   - Did you stumble but make it look intentional? That's definitely a win

3. **Collect Your Wins**:

   - Keep a "victory log" of your accomplishments

   - Take progress photos

- Document your journey

- Save those memories for when your confidence needs a boost

The Battle Scars Philosophy

My wrists don't look like normal wrists anymore. Neither do my shoulders. Or a lot of other parts of me, thanks to years of pushing limits. I used to try to hide these permanent alterations to my body. Now? I wear my battle scars like badges of honor. Because true confidence isn't about being perfect—it's about being perfectly okay with your imperfections.

The Mirror Task (No Escape)

Here's a simple way to boost your confidence every morning:

1. Stand in front of a mirror

2. Look yourself in the eye

3. Say something positive about yourself

4. Try not to get distracted by wondering if you've always had that little freckle

(Bonus points if you flex while doing this. Extra bonus points if someone walks in on you mid-pose.)

Real-Life Examples of Confidence Building

Remember that time I had to redesign my entire routine four weeks before competition because of a blown ACL? That wasn't confidence—that was pure stubbornness masked as confidence. But here's the thing: sometimes you have to fake it until you make it.

Or how about the time I competed with a broken leg and won? That wasn't confidence either—that was determination with a side of "Well, this is happening." But each time I pushed through something scary or difficult, my confidence grew.

Whitney's Go-To Confidence Boosters

1. **Power Songs**:
   Pick music that makes you feel like a superhero
   (Bring on my favorite Hip-Hop)

2. **Power Outfit**:
   Wear something that makes you feel unstoppable
   (Preferably something that won't malfunction mid-activity)

3. **Motivational Quote**:
   Find one that resonates with you
   (Mine is "You don't HAVE to, you GET to")

4. **Secret Weapon**:
   Have something that always makes you feel confident
   (Think about your most unique skill or a stupid human trick)

Your Turn: Build Your Confidence Arsenal

This week, try:

1. Doing one thing that scares you (within reason)

2. Celebrating one small win each day

3. Writing down your victories

4. Lean into your "I Am" statements—model those characteristics each day

Remember: Confidence isn't about never falling—it's about knowing you can get back up, and keep going. Even if you have to improvise the whole thing.

Because at the end of the day, true confidence comes from knowing that no matter what life throws at you—whether it's a broken bone, a wardrobe malfunction, or an accidental emoji rebellion—you can handle it.

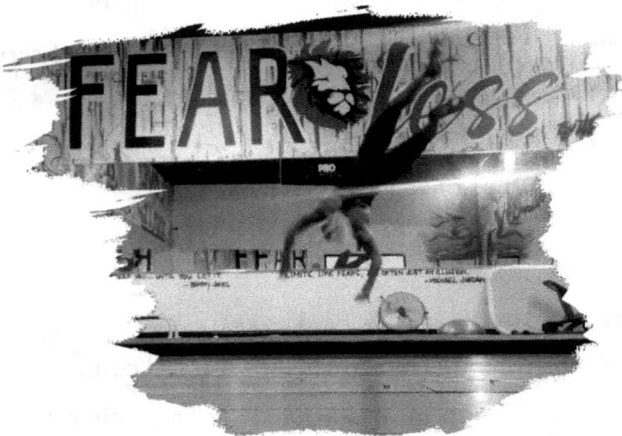

Your Turn:

What's one thing you're proud of pushing through this week, and how will you use that win to fuel your next challenge?

_____
_____
_____
_____
_____
_____
_____
_____
_____
_____
_____
_____
_____

What's the toughest thing you faced and conquered recently? Break down exactly how you did it.

_____

_____

_____

_____

_____

_____

_____

_____

_____

_____

_____

_____

_____

_____

_____

_____

_____

_____

_____

_____

_____

_____

_____

CHAPTER 17

Bonus: Behind the Scenes of Win Broken

What It Really Means to Win Broken

"Win broken" isn't just a catchy phrase—it's my life philosophy. It's about showing up when life feels messy, chaotic, and imperfect. It's about embracing your cracks, your flaws, and your struggles, and deciding that they don't define you—they refine you.

I've had 18 surgeries (and counting—because apparently, I'm collecting them like some people collect stamps), broken almost every bone in my body, and somehow managed to raise two amazing boys as a single mom while building businesses and chasing world titles.

The Reality Behind the Pages

People see me on stage at competitions and think I've got it all figured out—this polished, professional athlete who never misses a beat. Oh, if they only knew! They don't see the time my hair extension made an unscheduled appearance during a live TV interview, stubbornly refusing to detach from my hand mid-interview. Or the time I got the uncontrollable hiccups during a major meeting with the Diamondbacks and turned what should have been a serious meeting into an impromptu comedy show.

That's exactly what this book is about—the beautiful chaos behind the highlight reel. Those real, raw moments when you're caught between laughing and crying, so you end up doing both while trying to maintain some dignity. Like trying to pull off The Rock's signature eyebrow raise and grin but failing spectacularly. (Spoiler alert: I can't do it either, but hey, at least my failed attempts have provided endless entertainment for my boys and friends.)

The Writing Process: A New Kind of Challenge

Some days, writing was like trying to do a backflip for the first time—scary, exciting, and a real possibility of landing on your face. There were days when I thought:

- "Maybe I should just stick to flipping"

- "Can I tell these stories without embarrassing myself?"

- "Will people understand why I sometimes reset my own broken bones?"

- "Should I mention the time I accidentally posted middle finger emojis instead of pointing fingers?"

(Spoiler alert: I decided to tell it all because, hey, authenticity means embracing your fails as much as your wins.)

Lessons Learned Along the Way

Writing about my journey made me realize a few things:

1. **Every Struggle Has Value**:

   Even the embarrassing moments, like that spelling bee zipper incident, teach us something. (In that case, always check your fly and maybe don't wear cheap jeans to important events.)

2. **Humor Heals**:

   Sometimes the best way to battle through pain is to find the funny side. Like when I broke my nose and saw it as a free alignment opportunity. (Again, please don't try this at home.)

3. **Community Matters**:

   We're all a little broken, but together we're unbreakable. Unless we try to build a human pyramid in plank position—then all bets are off.

The Messages I Hope You Take Away

If you're reading this book and thinking, "Wow, this Whitney person is a hot mess," you're not wrong. But here's what I want you to remember:

1. You don't have to be perfect to be powerful

2. Your struggles can become your strengths

3. It's okay to laugh at yourself

4. Sometimes the best routines are the ones you improvise

5. Always wear good underwear (because you never know when your going to high kick and split your pants)

What's Next?

Life is a continuous journey of growth, challenges, and occasional wardrobe malfunctions. As I wrap up this book, I'm already thinking about what's next. More competitions? Maybe. More adventures? Most definitely. More opportunities to face-plant gracefully in front of live audiences? Probably inevitable.

But that's the beauty of winning broken—there's always another chapter to write, another challenge to face, and another opportunity to show up and say, "Watch this!" (Followed immediately by "Okay, that didn't go as planned, but check out my next trick!")

Your Turn to Win Broken

As you close this book, remember:

- Your struggles don't define you

- Your response to challenges do

- Your imperfections make you interesting

- Your recovery game can be stronger than your perfect performance

- Your story is still being written

Final Thoughts

Writing this book has felt a lot like performing one of my wild and crazy routines—complete with unexpected twists, moments of doubt, but with fewer injuries and way more home-baked cookies. And here's what I've learned: sometimes the most powerful stories aren't about the perfect landing—they're about what happens when the landing goes sideways and you somehow turn it into a signature move.

Because at the end of the day, winning broken isn't about having it all together—it's about embracing every crack, scar, and stumble along the way. It's about getting up one more time than you fall, laughing a little harder than you cry, and maybe—just maybe—inspiring someone else to own their story, battle wounds and all.

Now go out there and win broken. And if you fall? Make it look intentional. Trust me, I'm an expert at that part.

Your Turn:

What's your 'behind the scenes' story - the one that shows who you really are when no one's watching?

_____

_____

_____

_____

_____

_____

_____

_____

_____

_____

_____

_____

_____

_____

What struggle are you facing that could become someone else's inspiration?

_____

_____

_____

_____

_____

_____

_____

_____

_____

_____

_____

_____

_____

_____

_____

_____

_____

_____

_____

_____

_____

_____

_____

_____

_____

Liz Freeman: Finding Joy in the Journey

Liz's story isn't your typical transformation tale. She didn't come to me as a competitive athlete or a mom looking to get back in shape. Instead, Liz came with a clear goal: to lose 40 pounds before she turned 40. At the time, she was dealing with a sleep disorder and lifestyle challenges that had left her feeling unhealthy and stuck.

What made Liz stand out was her determination. Even though hitting the gym was the last thing she wanted to do, she showed up. Every. Single. Time. When we began working together, Liz approached each workout as something she *had to* do—a chore on her to-do list. That's when I introduced her to my **H2G2 philosophy**: shifting from a mindset of "have to" to "get to."

At first, Liz was skeptical. But as the weeks went on, something began to shift. She started to see each session not as an obligation, but as an opportunity—a chance to take back control of her health and her life. That simple change in perspective turned workouts from a burden into a privilege, and she began embracing every step of her journey with renewed energy.

As her health improved, her personality began to shine. Beneath the exhaustion was a vibrant soul with a laugh so contagious it could light up the whole gym. Our sessions went from "blood, sweat, and tears" to "blood, sweat, and uncontrollable giggles." She brought an energy that was absolutely electric.

Not only did Liz hit her goal of losing 40 pounds by her 40th birthday, but she didn't stop there. She kept setting new goals and smashing them, proving to herself just how much she was capable of achieving. Every milestone reinforced her *get to* mindset—she wasn't just working out to lose weight anymore; she was discovering what it felt like to truly take care of herself.

Her transformation didn't stop at physical changes. Liz's newfound energy and confidence spilled into every area of her life. She gained clarity in her career, strengthened her drive, and enriched her social life. The best part? Her partner, inspired by Liz's incredible progress, decided to start their own fitness journey. Now, they're both making this not just a phase, but a lifestyle they share together.

Liz didn't just get healthier—she rediscovered her joy. She found her voice. And she fully embraced the **H2G2 philosophy**, transforming obligations into opportunities and turning her life around. Her story proves that the greatest victory isn't just about reaching your goals but about discovering who you truly are when you feel strong enough to let your light shine through.

That's the thing about transformation—when you commit to showing up for yourself, you never know how many lives you'll end up touching along the way.

Closing

You've Got This—Now Go Win Broken

"EYES FORWARD. MIND FOCUSED. HEART READY.
GAME ON, WORLD"

B y now, you've read about my various face plants (both literal and metaphorical), wardrobe malfunctions that would make a reality show blush, and that time I casually put my own shoulder back in place during the Olympia because, well, the show must go on. You've probably either thought "This woman is inspiring" or "This woman is crazy." Plot twist: it's probably a little bit of both.

Here's the truth: *Win Broken* isn't about having it all together. It's about showing up when life feels messy, when progress feels slow, and when your costume decides to stage a rebellion mid-performance. It's about finding the cracks, the imperfections, and the struggles—and deciding to shine through them anyway.

Remember: perfection is boring. It's unattainable. But showing up as your beautifully imperfect self? That's where the magic happens. That's where you grow. That's where you win.

The Lessons We've Learned Together

Let's recap some key takeaways:

- You don't HAVE to, you GET to

- Sometimes your biggest setbacks lead to your greatest comebacks

- Your battle scars are badges of honor

- Always check your costume fit

- Double-check your emojis before posting

- Maybe let professionals handle the broken bones (do as I say, not as I do)

Your Next Steps: Your Win Broken Plan

Here's your mission, should you choose to accept it:

1. **Set Your First Goal:**

   What's one thing you want to achieve in the next 30 days? Write it down. Make it specific. And commit to it—even if it scares you a little. (Just maybe avoid hungry lions.)

2. **Find Your Why**:

Dig deep. Why does this goal matter? What will it change for you? Let that be your anchor when things get tough or when your metaphorical bikini pops mid-routine.

3. **Take One Step Today**:

Don't wait until Monday, or next month, or when Mercury isn't in retrograde. Start now. Take one small action that moves you closer to your goal.

4. **Celebrate Every Win**:

No matter how small, celebrate every step forward. Progress deserves recognition—even if that progress is simply, "I didn't break any fingernails doing push-ups today."

Your Story Isn't Over

Here's the best part: this isn't the end of your story. It's just the beginning. Wherever you are right now—whether you're just starting out, in the middle of a messy season, or ready to take things to the next level—you're exactly where you're supposed to be.

Keep going. Keep laughing. Keep getting back up. Keep exuding confidence. Keep doing whatever it takes to *win broken*.

And remember: you don't have to do it perfectly. You just have to do it authentically, with whatever mix of grace and chaos you bring to the table. Because sometimes the most powerful thing you can do is embrace your struggles, own your story, and maybe add some jazz hands for good measure.

If you ever need a reminder, pick up this book, flip to any page, and know that somewhere out there, I'm probably either:

a) Attempting something slightly crazy

b) Recovering from attempting something slightly crazy

c) Planning my next slightly crazy attempt

d) All of the above

Because that's how you win broken—not letting fear, failure, or a few face plants stop you from living your fullest life.

You've got this. You've had it all along. Now go out there and win broken—in your own messy but magical way.

And if anyone tries to tell you you can't? Just smile and say, "Watch me."

(Just maybe have a backup plan ready. And good underwear. Always good underwear.)

#WIN BROKEN

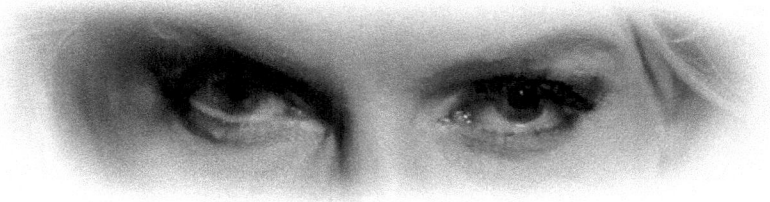

Your Turn:

Looking at your biggest challenge right now: How will you win broken? What's your first step forward, and what will make this story worth telling later?

_____

_____

_____

_____

_____

_____

_____

_____

_____

_____

_____

_____

What's your win broken story going to be? Map out your first three steps.

_____

_____

_____

_____

_____

_____

_____

_____

_____

_____

_____

_____

_____

_____

_____

_____

_____

_____

_____

_____

_____

_____

_____

_____

_____

Appendix A: Goal-Setting Worksheet

Your Win Broken Action Plan

Step 1: Define Your Goal

What do you want to achieve? Be specific and write it down:

- My goal is: _____

- Target date: _____

- This goal matters because: _____

Step 2: Find Your Why

Using the Why Ladder (ask "why" 5 times):

1. Why do I want this? _____

2. Why does that matter? _____

3. Why is that important? _____

4. Why would that make a difference? _____

5. Why is that my deepest motivation? _____

Step 3: Break It Down

List 3 smaller steps that will move you toward your goal:

    1.

    2.

    3.

Step 4: Identify Potential Obstacles

What might get in your way?

- Obstacle 1: _____
  Solution: _____

- Obstacle 2: _____
  Solution: _____

- Obstacle 3: _____
  Solution: _____

Step 5: Create Your Support System

Who can help you achieve this goal?

- Accountability partner: _____

- Mentor/Coach: _____

- Cheerleaders: _____

Step 6: Track Your Progress

Weekly check-in points:

- Week 1 Progress: _____

- Week 2 Progress: _____

- Week 3 Progress: _____

- Week 4 Progress: _____

Step 7: Celebration Plan

How will you celebrate your:

- Small wins: _____

- Milestones: _____

- Final achievement: _____

Remember:

- Progress over perfection

- You don't HAVE to, you GET to

- Every setback is setting you up for a comeback

- Your struggles can become your strengths

Weekly Reflection

What went well? _____

What did I learn? _____

How did I overcome challenges? _____

What am I proud of? _____

What needs adjustment? _____

Monthly Review

Looking back:

- Biggest victory: _____

- Most valuable lesson: _____

- Proudest moment: _____

- Next month's focus: _____

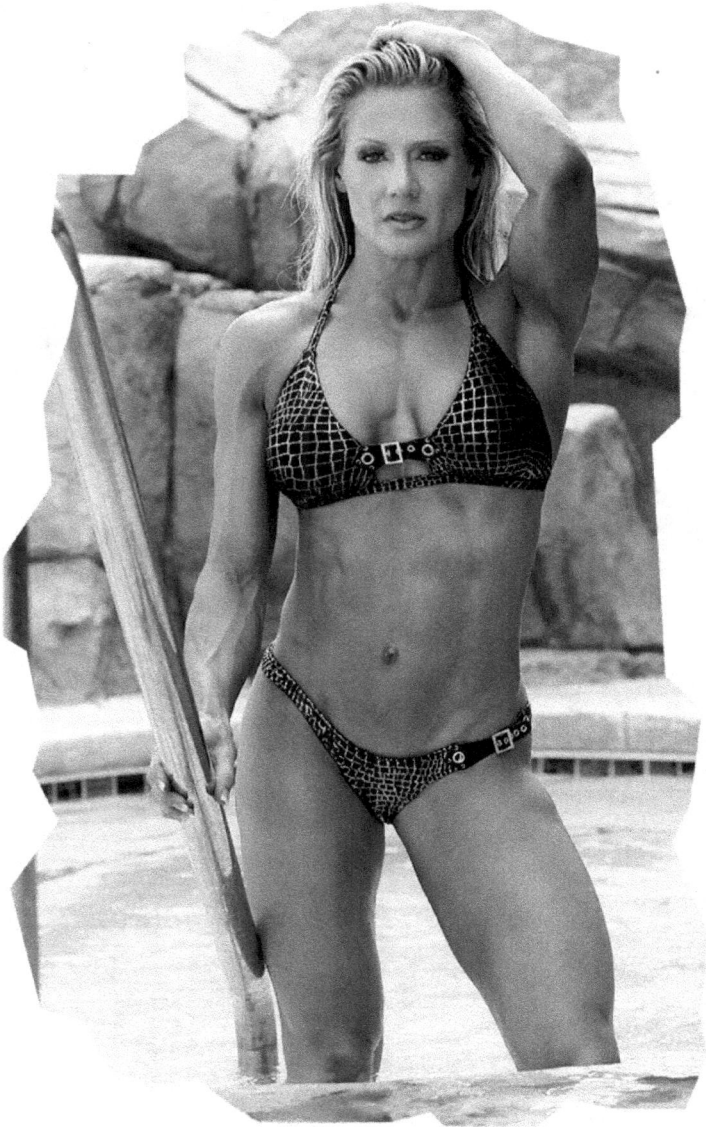

Appendix B:

30-Day Win Broken Challenge

Ready to put the win broken philosophy into action? Here's your 30-day roadmap to building unstoppable momentum. Remember: it's not about being perfect—it's about showing up and making progress.

Week 1: Building Your Foundation

Day 1-7: Mindset Reset

- Day 1: Write your "I GET to" list (replace "have to" with "get to")

- Day 2: Set your big goal and identify your "why"

- Day 3: Share your goal with an accountability partner

- Day 4: Create your morning power routine

- Day 5: Face one small fear (Maybe post your goal on social media with **#WinBroken**)

- Day 6: Document your first week's journey

- Day 7: Celebrate your first week (yes, already!)

Week 2: Taking Action

Day 8-14: Building Momentum

- Day 8: Try something new in your workout

- Day 9: Practice your recovery pose (trust me, you'll use it)

- Day 10: Connect with someone who inspires you

- Day 11: Step outside your comfort zone

- Day 12: Document a small win

- Day 13: Learn from a setback

- Day 14: Review and reset for week 3

Week 3: Pushing Boundaries

Day 15-21: Leveling Up

- Day 15: Double down on your main goal

- Day 16: Help someone else win broken

- Day 17: Face a bigger fear

- Day 18: Create your power playlist

- Day 19: Practice resilience

- Day 20: Share your progress story

- Day 21: Celebrate your progress (dancing encouraged)

Week 4: Becoming Unstoppable

Day 22-30: Finishing Strong

- Day 22: Increase your challenge level

- Day 23: Inspire someone else

- Day 24: Document your transformation

- Day 25: Plan your next big goal

- Day 26: Face your biggest fear yet

- Day 27: Share your success strategy

- Day 28: Create your victory dance

- Day 29: Plan your celebration

- Day 30: Reflect and reset for what's next

Daily Must-Dos:

1. Start each day with gratitude

2. Document one win (no matter how small)

3. Strike a power pose

4. End each day with reflection

Remember:

- Progress over perfection

- Every setback is temporary

- Your struggles make you stronger

- Keep your sense of humor

- Celebrate everything

Tracking Your Progress:

Use the Goal-Setting Worksheet (Appendix A) to track your daily progress and wins. Remember to:

- Note your daily victories

- Document your challenges and how you overcame them

- Track your energy levels

- Record your mood

- List your proud moments

Bonus Challenges:

- Create your own recovery pose

- Make someone else laugh

- Try something that scares you (within reason)

- Share your journey with others

- Help someone else overcome their fear

Remember: This challenge isn't about being perfect—it's about progress, persistence, and maybe a few wonderfully imperfect moments along the way. Now go out there and show the world what it looks like to win broken!

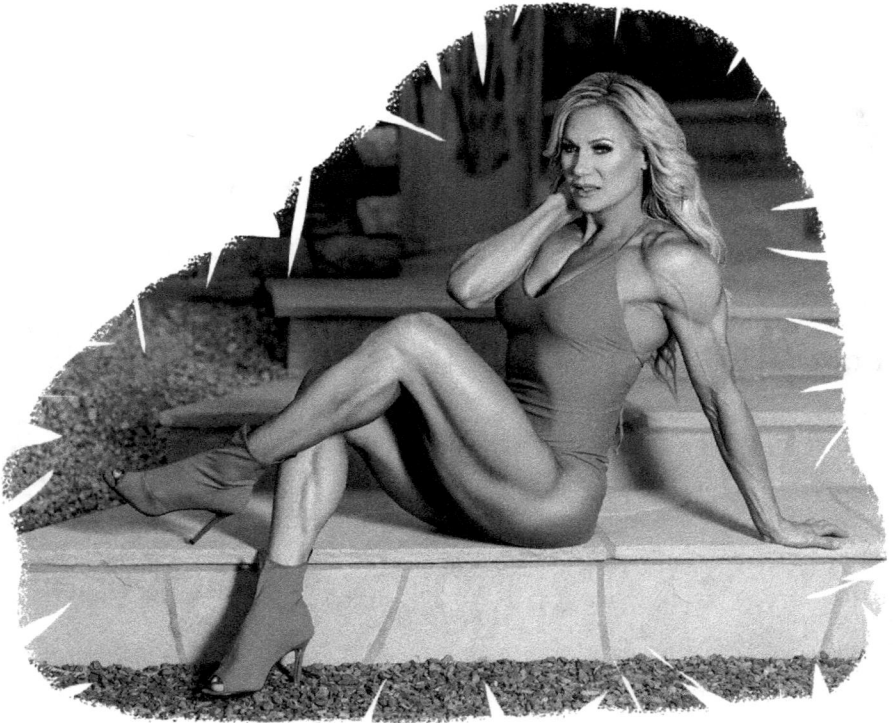

APPENDIX C:

Whitney's Winning Playlist

When you need that extra push, here's what gets me fired up and ready to take on anything. These aren't just songs—they're the soundtrack to help me win broken:

1. "Legends Are Made" - Sam Tinnesz

2. "Don't Stop Believin'" - Journey

3. "Run for Cover" - Phantom Passenger, King Green

4. "Unstoppable" - Sia

5. "Till I Collapse" - Eminem

6. "Hall of Fame" - The Script, will.i.am

7. "Big Dawgs" - Humankind, Kalmi

8. "Bring Em Out" - T.I.

9. "Lose Yourself" - Eminem

10. "Thunderstruck" - AC/DC

11. "Turn Down For What" - DJ Snake, Lil Jon

12. "All I Do Is Win" - DJ Khaled, T-Pain, Ludacris

Photo Credits:

Front Cover:

Lion Face Photo Credit - *Lauren Henry*

Leaping Photo Credit – *Herman Diviri*

Part 1 – *Sean Nelson*

Page 10 – *Body Photage*

Page 13 – *George Kontaxis*

Page 37 – *J.M. Manion*

Page 43 – *Kai York*

Page 67 – *Tony Brown*

Page 92 – *Quan Phu*

Page 99 – *George Kontaxis*

Page 105 – *Nick Sorenson*

Page 112 – *Herman Diviri*

Page 115 – *Kai York*

Page 131 – *Doug Scalia*

Page 137 – *Rob Pic Photography*

Page 185 – *Isaac Hinds*

Page 192 – *Sean Nelson*

Page 195 – *Sean Nelson*

About the Author – *George Kontaxis*

Back Cover – *Chris Nicoll*

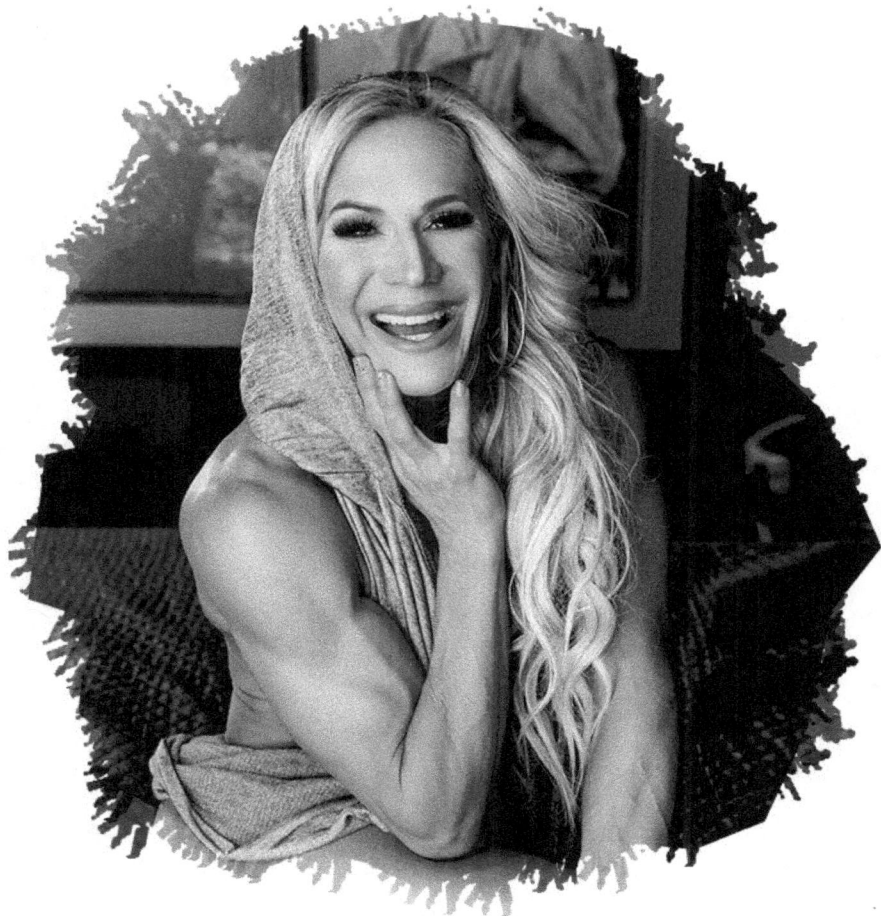

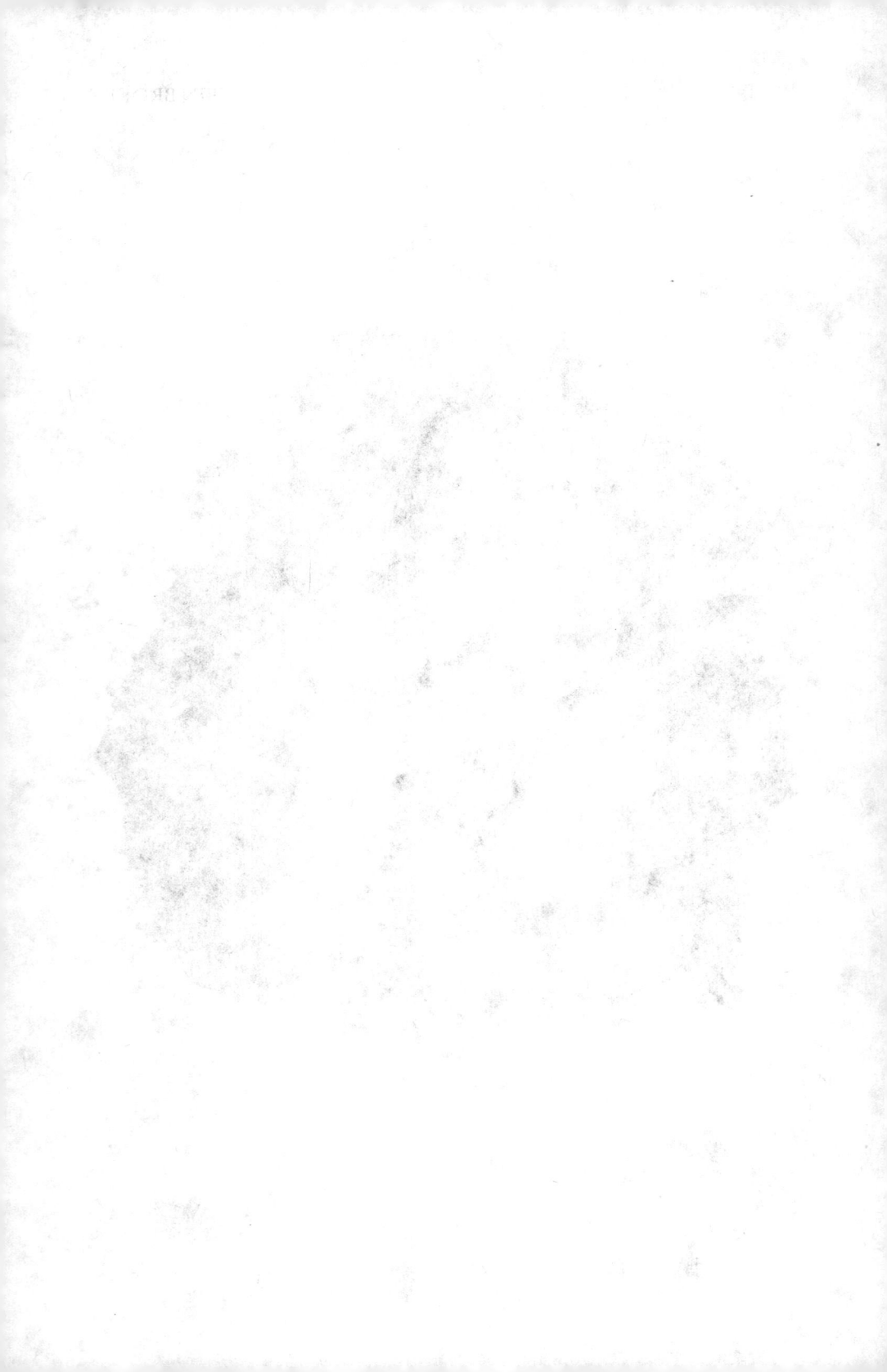

Acknowledgements

Writing this book has been a journey of challenges, learning, and growth—one that would not have been possible without the unwavering support of some truly remarkable individuals.

First and foremost, to my boys, Brody and Jake: you are my world, my everything. Thank you for filling life with laughter, energy, and spontaneity. Your endless love, late-night laughter, and playful teasing of my quirks kept me grounded and reminded me to embrace the joy in the process. You inspire me daily to stay humble, dream big, remain curious, and never take life too seriously.

To Sway, thank you for your countless pep talks, brainstorming ideas, never-ending patience, and your willingness to read "just one more draft." You've been a part of so many life events, and your unique ability to bring laughter to heavy moments is a gift I deeply appreciate. While this book may bear my name, it's powered by you and the boys. Thank you for encouraging me to share more of myself than I ever thought I would.

To my best friends—Tiana Zang, Sally Williams, and Ashley Garcia: Tiana, our story began before we did, with two mothers who became friends and dreamed their daughters would share the same bond. They got their wish. From our first breaths to this day, we've been absolutely inseparable—you're my soul sister, carrying forward a legacy of friendship that started with the women who raised us. Sally and Ashley, our shared passions brought us together as adults, but it's all of our wild personalities (amplified by Tiana's rowdiness) that have kept us all close. True friends don't just celebrate your successes; they challenge you to achieve them. The unwavering support from you three throughout this journey has meant the world to me.

To my mentor and friend, Joe Polish: your wisdom and advice have been an invaluable source of motivation. Your belief in me gave me the confidence to see this project through.

And to Dave Streen: you deserve an Olympia Trophy—or at the very least, a lifetime supply of coffee—for your patience and guidance. Thank you for helping me turn my messy ideas into something coherent and, hopefully, entertaining.

This book is a labor of love, and it would not have been possible without each of you. From the bottom of my heart, thank you.

Let's Connect

Please send everyone you know to **WhitneysBook.com**

(If you loved this book—I'd love for you to leave a review)

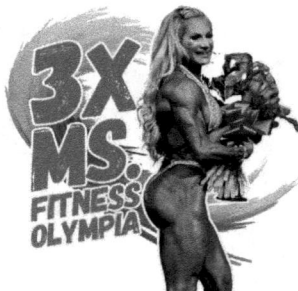

Website: **EmpoweringLegends.com**

Website: **FitWhitJones.com**

Email: **FitWhitJones@gmail.com**

Instagram: **@whitneyjones_ifbbpro**

Facebook: facebook.com/**WhitneyEstesJones**

Facebook Fan Page: facebook.com/**WhitneyJonesFitnessPro**

LinkedIn: **@3xmsolympiawhitneyjones**

TikTok: **@whitneyjonespro**

YouTube: **@WhitneyJonesPro**

Twitter: **@WhitneyJonesAZ**

About the Author

Whitney Jones is a force of nature who proves that life's greatest challenges often become our greatest opportunities. As a three-time Ms. Fitness Olympia Champion and the Arnold Classic Ms. Fitness International winner, Whitney didn't discover fitness competitions until her early 30s—proving it's never too late to chase extraordinary dreams.

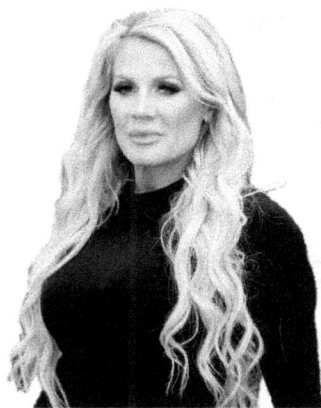

Known for her infectious energy and unapologetic authenticity, Whitney has transformed countless lives through her coaching programs, speaking engagements, and signature "Win Broken" philosophy. Her journey from single mom facing adversity to becoming a world champion athlete has inspired thousands to push past their perceived limitations. In 2018, she claimed her first world championship title at the Arnold Classic Ms. Fitness International while competing with a torn ACL—months after recovering from neck surgery.

Despite having a body that's been literally pieced back together (including a 12-piece metal cage in her neck and 18 surgeries), Whitney continues to defy expectations and break barriers in the fitness industry. She's appeared on numerous fitness magazine covers, been featured in leading publications, and has built a global community of individuals committed to winning broken.

Through her transformative platform which you can find at **EmpoweringLegends.com**, Whitney helps people all over the world discover their inner strength and build unstoppable confidence. Her innovative coaching methods combine practical strategies with an emphasis on finding joy and humor in life's challenges, proving that grit and grace can coexist on the path to success.

When she's not coaching clients, or running her businesses, you'll find Whitney dancing in her car at stoplights, hunting down the perfect donut, or creating chaos-filled adventures with her two boys. She believes in living life full-out, finding joy in the journey, and never letting your circumstances dictate your destiny.

Whitney resides in Arizona, where she continues to expand her impact through mentorship and coaching programs, speaking engagements, and now this book—her raw and real guide to turning life's challenges into your greatest victories.

For more information about Whitney's programs and speaking engagements, visit **FitWhitJones.com** or follow her on her social media platforms to connect.

EMPOWERING LEGENDS
Ready to Become Legendary?

You've made it this far. You've read about resilience, breakthroughs, setbacks turned into comebacks, and the power hidden within life's toughest moments. But reading about transformation is just the beginning.

Now it's your turn.

At Empowering Legends, we've built something extraordinary—a place where your struggles become strengths, and your setbacks fuel your greatest triumphs. A community where:

- You're supported by people who understand your journey

- Every challenge is transformed into an opportunity

- Victories, big or small, are celebrated together

- Real strategies turn inspiration into action

This where mindset meets mastery, courage meets community, and "I can't" transforms into "Watch me."

Why Join Right Now?

Because you're ready. You feel it—the drive, the spark, the voice inside telling you that you're meant for more. Listen to it.

At **Empowering Legends** you'll experience:

- Powerful daily inspiration that moves you forward

- Practical tools you can apply immediately

- A community dedicated to your growth and success

- Authentic connections and unwavering support

Here's What to Do:

- Close this book (yeah, we actually said that!)

- Go to EmpoweringLegends.com

- Become part of our empowering community

- Take the first step to becoming legendary

Don't wait for Monday. Don't wait until you're "ready." Don't wait until things are perfect.

If you've learned anything, it's that perfect isn't necessary—but stepping forward is everything.

Instead of one day, make this *Day One!*

Visit **EmpoweringLegends.com** now.

It's your time to rise. Let's become legends together.

See you inside!

– Whitney

Scan me!

Can't wait to see you on the inside! **EmpoweringLegends.com**

WRITE YOUR OWN BOOK

Books Build Brands. Let's Begin Yours!

Want to turn your expertise into a published book? WeHelpAuthors.com specializes in taking you from idea to published author.

Our team provides everything you need:

- Book Planning & Strategy

- Writing & Editing

- Design & Formatting

- Publishing & Marketing

Visit **WeHelpAuthors.com** or email support@wehelpauthors.com to start your author journey today.

www.ingramcontent.com/pod-product-compliance
Lightning Source LLC
Chambersburg PA
CBHW052127270326
41930CB00012B/2784